Companion for
3rd MBBS

Companion for 3rd MBBS

Thirteenth Edition

Singi Yatiraj
Kalaburagi, Karnataka
India

Co-author
Roopali Somani
Kalaburagi, Karnataka
India

JAYPEE

JAYPEE BROTHERS MEDICAL PUBLISHERS
The Health Sciences Publisher
New Delhi | London

Jaypee Brothers Medical Publishers (P) Ltd

Headquarters
Jaypee Brothers Medical Publishers (P) Ltd
4838/24, Ansari Road, Daryaganj
New Delhi 110 002, India
Phone: +91-11-43574357
Fax: +91-11-43574314
Email: jaypee@jaypeebrothers.com

Overseas Office
J.P. Medical Ltd
83 Victoria Street, London
SW1H 0HW (UK)
Phone: +44 20 3170 8910
Fax: +44 (0)20 3008 6180
Email: info@jpmedpub.com

Website: www.jaypeebrothers.com
Website: www.jaypeedigital.com

Companion for 3rd MBBS

First Edition	:	*2007*	*Eighth Edition*	:	*2015*
Second Edition	:	*2008*	*Ninth Edition*	:	*2016*
Third Edition	:	*2009*	*Tenth Edition*	:	*2017*
Fourth Edition	:	*2010*	*Eleventh Edition*	:	*2018*
Fifth Edition	:	*2011*	*Twelfth Edition*	:	*2019*
Sixth Edition	:	*2012*	*Thirteenth Edition*	:	**2020**
Seventh Edition	:	*2014*			

ISBN 978-93-89776-50-8

Printed at

| | ॐ श्री फलौदी ब्रम्हाणी देवी नमः | |

Om Shri Falaudi Brahmani Devi Namah

Dedicated to

That person
Who has brought happiness in my life
Who has given me a reason to smile
Who has trusted me all the time and
Showed me that I can do it.

This book is a tribute to my
Late Sister Anupama
and
Grandmother Rajubai

Preface

Companion series has been a huge success among the medical students of Karnataka. Very sincere and heartfelt thanks to all my loyal readers for making it the most preferred question bank in comparison to other question banks.

It is my promise to deliver the latest questions of the Rajiv Gandhi University of Health Sciences (RGUHS), Karnataka, India, in their original format with cross-reference to the latest editions of the student-popular undergraduate books. And, I take liberty to consider your unabated support for these titles.

I sincerely solicit your valuable comments in this regard. So please do write your comments to *singi_yatiraj@yahoo.com* or *@facebook.*

Wishing you all the best.

Singi Yatiraj
www.drsingiyatiraj.5u.com

Acknowledgments

I would like to thank:

- Dr B Mallikarjun, Former Dean, MR Medical College, Kalaburagi, Karnataka, India, for his encouragement and support.
- All the staff members and postgraduates, Department of Community Medicine, Ophthalmology and Otorhinolaryngology, MR Medical College, Kalaburagi, for their selfless excellent teaching.
- My teachers, for they are the ones who made me this capable.
- My friends Kiran, Nagaraj and Wali, for their help, support, suggestions and encouragement throughout the project.
- Mr Kalburgi and *Late* Sri Puranik of Computer Section, for providing me the question papers of the university examinations.
- All the students who have helped me compile the question bank.
- Mr Md Bari, Mr Yousuf Patel and Mr Rashid, Star Computers, for all the assistance in timely and neat computer printing of the manuscript.
- Mr Suresh Prithvi, Proprietor, M/s Prithvi Book Agency and his staff, for their support, cooperation and promoting this title. Mr Santosh Patil, Proprietor, M/s SS Patil Book Sellers and staff, for their cooperation.
- My all friends and well-wishers, for their best wishes.
- Shri Jitendar P Vij (Group Chairman), Mr Ankit Vij (Managing Director), and Mr MS Mani (Group President) of M/s Jaypee Brothers Medical Publishers (P) Ltd, New Delhi, India, for publishing the book in the same format as wanted well in time.
- Mr Venugopal (Associate Director–South) and other staff members of Jaypee Brothers, Bengaluru Branch, for taking this book to every corner of Karnataka.
- Dr Madhu Choudhary (Associate Director—Content Strategy), Ms Pooja Bhandari (Production Head), Ms Sunita Katla (Executive Assistant to Group Chairman and Publishing Manager), Ms Samina Khan (Executive Assistant to Publishing Head—Education), Mr Rajesh Sharma (Production Coordinator), Ms Seema Dogra (Cover Visualizer), Ms Uma Adhikari, Mr Laxmidhar Padhiary, and others at the M/s Jaypee Brothers Medical Publishers (P) Ltd, New Delhi, for their painstaking effort to make this book attractive and lucid.
- All the students, for their overwhelming response and support to my prior endeavors.

- All those who have helped me directly or indirectly.
- Most important of all, my parents, sister, uncles and aunties, for their eternal love, care and support.
- Above all, Dr Roopali Somani, my cousin for helping me out with page numbering of new papers.

Thank you all of you,

Without you, this book would not have been a reality.

Contents

COMMUNITY MEDICINE

1. Man and Medicine: Towards Health for All 11
2. Concept of Health and Disease 11
3. Principles of Epidemiologic Methods 16
4. Screening for Disease 24
5. Epidemiology of Communicable Diseases 25
   A. Respiratory Infections 25
   B. Intestinal Infections 28
   C. Arthropod-borne Infections 31
   D. Zoonoses 33
   E. Surface Infections 35
   F. Emerging and Re-emerging Infectious Diseases 37
   G. Hospital-acquired Infections 37
6. Epidemiology of Chronic Noncommunicable Diseases and Conditions 38
7. Health Programs in India 42
8. Millennium Development Goals to Sustainable Development Goals 46
9. Demography and Family Planning 46
10. Preventive Medicine in Obstetrics, Pediatrics and Geriatrics 50
11. Nutrition and Health 57
12. Social Science and Health 62
13. Environment and Health 65
14. Hospital Waste Management 71
15. Disaster Management 72
16. Occupational Health 73
17. Genetics and Health 76
18. Mental Health 77
19. Health Information and Basic Medical Statistics 78
20. Communication for Health Education 81
21. Health Planning and Management 83
22. Health Care of the Community 86
23. International Health 89

OPHTHALMOLOGY

Section I: Anatomy and Physiology of the Eye

1. Anatomy and Development of the Eye 102
2. Physiology of Eye and Vision 102

Section II: Optics and Refraction

3. Elementary and Physiological Optics 102
4. Errors of Refraction and Accommodation 102

Section III: Diseases of Eye and Ocular Adnexa

5. Diseases of Conjunctiva 104
6. Diseases of Cornea 107
7. Diseases of Sclera 110
8. Diseases of Uveal Tract 111
9. Diseases of Lens 113
10. Glaucoma 117
11. Diseases of Vitreous 120
12. Diseases of Retina 120
13. Neuro-ophthalmology 122
14. Disorders of Ocular Motility 125
15. Diseases of Eyelids 126
16. Diseases of Lacrimal Apparatus 128
17. Diseases of Orbit 130
18. Ocular Injuries 131

Section IV: Ocular Therapeutics

19. Ocular Pharmacology 133
20. Lasers and Cryotherapy in Ophthalmology 135

Section V: Systemic and Community Ophthalmology

21. Systemic OphthalmologY 135
22. Community Ophthalmology 136

Section VI: Practical Ophthalmology

23. Clinical Methods in Ophthalmology 137
24. Clinical Ophthalmic Cases 140
25. Darkroom Procedures 140
26. Ophthalmic Instruments and Operative Ophthalmology 140

OTORHINOLARYNGOLOGY

Section I: Diseases of Ear

1. Anatomy of Ear 150
2. Peripheral Receptors and Physiology of Auditory and Vestibular System 151
3. Audiology and Acoustics 151
4. Assessment of Hearing 151
5. Hearing Loss 152
6. Assessment of Vestibular Functions 154
7. Disorders of Vestibular System 154
8. Diseases of External Ear 154
9. Eustachian Tube and its Disorders 156
10. Disorders of Middle Ear 156
11. Cholesteatoma and Chronic Suppurative Otitis Media 157
12. Complications of Otitis Media 158
13. Otosclerosis 159
14. Facial Nerve and its Disorders 160
15. Meniere's Disease 161
16. Tumors of External Ear 161
17. Tumors of Middle Ear and Mastoid 161
18. Acoustic Neuroma 162
19. The Deaf Child 162
20. Rehabilitation of the Hearing Impaired 162
21. Otalgia (Earache) 162
22. Tinnitus 163

Section II: Diseases of Nose and Paranasal Sinuses

23. Anatomy of Nose 163
24. Physiology of Nose 164
25. Diseases of External Nose and Nasal Vestibule 164
26. Nasal Septum and its Diseases 165
27. Acute and Chronic Rhinitis 165
28. Granulomatous Diseases of Nose 166
29. Miscellaneous Disorders of Nasal Cavity 167
30. Allergic Rhinitis 168
31. Vasomotor and Other Forms of Nonallergic Rhinitis 168
32. Nasal Polyp 168
33. Epistaxis 169
34. Trauma to the Face 170
35. Anatomy and Physiology of Paranasal Sinuses 171

36. Acute Sinusitis 171
37. Chronic Sinusitis 171
38. Complications of Sinusitis 172
39. Neoplasms of Nasal Cavity 172
40. Neoplasms of Paranasal Sinuses 173
41. Proptosis 173

Section III: Diseases of Oral Cavity and Salivary Glands

42. Anatomy of Oral Cavity 173
43. Common Disorders of Oral Cavity 173
44. Tumors of Oral Cavity 174
45. Non-neoplastic Disorders of Salivary Glands 174
46. Neoplasms of Salivary Glands 174

Section IV: Diseases of Pharynx

47. Anatomy and Physiology of Pharynx 175
48. Adenoids and Other Inflammations of Nasopharynx 175
49. Tumors of Nasopharynx 176
50. Acute and Chronic Pharyngitis 176
51. Acute and Chronic Tonsillitis 177
52. Head and Neck Space Infections 178
53. Tumors of Oropharynx 179
54. Tumors of the Hypopharynx and Pharyngeal Pouch 180
55. Snoring and Sleep Apnea 180

Section V: Diseases of Larynx and Trachea

56. Anatomy and Physiology of Larynx 180
57. Laryngotracheal Trauma 181
58. Acute and Chronic Inflammations of Larynx 181
59. Congenital Lesions of Larynx and Stridor 181
60. Laryngeal Paralysis 182
61. Benign Tumors of Larynx 183
62. Cancer Larynx 184
63. Voice and Speech Disorders 184
64. Tracheostomy and Other Procedures for Airway Management 185
65. Foreign Bodies in Air Passage 186

Section VI: Thyroid Gland and its Disorders

66. Thyroid Gland and its Disorders 186

Section VII: Diseases of Esophagus

67. Anatomy and Physiology of Esophagus 186
68. Disorders of Esophagus 186
69. Dysphagia 187
70. Foreign Bodies in Food Passage 187

Section VIII: Recent Advances

71. Laser Surgery, Radiofrequency Surgery, Hyperbaric Oxygen Therapy and Coblation 188
72. Cryosurgery 188
73. Radiotherapy in Head and Neck Cancer 188
74. Chemotherapy in Head and Neck Cancer 188
75. HIV Infections/AIDS and ENT Manifestations 188

Section IX: Clinical Methods in ENT and Neck Masses

76. Clinical Methods in ENT 189
77. Neck Masses 189

Section X: Operative Surgery

78. Myringotomy 190
79. Ear Surgery and Approaches 190
80. Cortical Mastoidectomy 190
81. Radical Mastoidectomy 191
82. Modified Radical Mastoidectomy 191
83. Myringoplasty 191
84. Proof Puncture (Antral Irrigation) 191
85. Intranasal Inferior Meatal Antrostomy 191
86. Caldwell-Luc Operation 192
87. Submucous Resection of Nasal Septum (SMR Operation) 192
88. Septoplasty 192
89. Diagnostic Nasal Endoscopy 192
90. Endoscopic Sinus Surgery 193
91. Direct Laryngoscopy 193
92. Bronchoscopy 193
93. Esophagoscopy 193
94. Tonsillectomy 193
95. Adenoidectomy 194
96. Radiology in ENT 194

1

Community Medicine

REFERENCES

1. K Park **(PARK)**: Park's Textbook of Preventive and Social Medicine, 25th Edition, M/s Banarsidas Bhanot Publishers, Jabalpur, ₹ 1400/-
2. AH Suryakantha **(SYKNT)**: Community Medicine with Recent Advances, 5th Edition, Jaypee Brothers Medical Publishers (P) Ltd., New Delhi, ₹ 1395/-.

COURSE CONTENTS

THEORY

I. Evolution of Public Health and Concepts of Health

Must Know

- Evolution of public health
- Definition of health, holistic concept of health, appreciation of health as a relative concept, determinants of health
- Characteristics of agent, host and environmental factors in health and disease and the multifactorial etiology of disease
- Understanding the natural history of disease and application, interventions at various levels of prevention with appropriate examples
- Indices used in measurement of health
- Health profile in India.

II. Environment and Health

Must Know

- Water
  - The concept of safe and wholesome water
  - The requirement of sanitary sources of water
  - Understanding the methods of purification of water on small scale and large scale
  - Various biological standards including World Health Organization (WHO) guidelines for third world countries
  - Principles and methods for assessing quality of water
- Sources, health hazards and control of environmental pollution
- Problems in the disposable of refuse, sullage, human excreta and sewage and its remedies
- Awareness of standards of housing and the effect of poor housing on health
- Role of vectors in the causation of diseases
- Identifying features and mode of transmission of vector-borne diseases.

Desirable to Know

- Methods of vector control with advantages and limitations of each
- Modes of action, dose and application cycle of commonly used insecticides and rodenticides.

III. Health Eduction

Must Know

- Communicate effectively with individuals, family and community using tools and techniques of information, education and communication. To do so, the students should know:
  - Principles of communication, methods and evaluation of health education and understand and apply adult education methods
  - Appreciate barriers of effective communication

- List various methods of health education with their advantages and disadvantages
- Select and use of appropriate media (simple audiovisual) for effective health education
- Practice of health education

- Use every opportunity for health education of the individual, family and the community.

IV. Nutrition and Dietetics

Must Know

- Common sources of various nutrients and special nutritional requirements according to age, sex, activity, physiological condition
- Nutritional assessment of individual, families and the community by selection and using appropriate methods such as anthropometry, clinical, dietary, laboratory techniques
- Plan and recommend a suitable diet for the individuals and families bearing in mind the local availability of foods, economic status, etc.
- Common nutritional disorders—protein-energy malnutrition, vitamin A deficiency, anemia, iodine deficiency diseases, fluorosis, food toxin disease and the control and management
- National programs in nutrition
- Nutritional surveillance, education and rehabilitation.

V. Occupational Health

Must Know

- Relate the history of symptoms with the specific occupation including agriculture
- Employees State Insurance (ESI) Scheme
- Identification of the physical, chemical, biological and social hazards to which workers are exposed to while working in a specific occupational environment
- Influence of physical factors like heat, humidity, cold, radiation and noise on the health of the individual and community
- General preventive measures against these diseases including accident prevention.

Desirable to Know

- Various legislation in relation to occupational health.

VI. Medical Sociology and Community Mental Health

Must Know

- Conduct of a clinico-social evaluation of the individual in relation to social, economic and cultural aspects, educational and residential background; attitude to health, disease and to health services, the individuals, families and communities
- Assessment of barriers to good health, recovery from sickness and to lead a socially and economically productive life

- Development of good doctor-patient and community relationship
- Identification of sociocultural factors related to the health and disease in the context of urban and rural societies
- Impact of urbanization of health and disease
- National mental health program.

Desirable to Know

- Community psychiatry.

VII. Fundamentals of Biostatistics

Must Know

- The scope and uses of biostatistics
- Collection of data, common sampling techniques, simple statistical method for the analysis, classification, interpretation and presentation of data, frequency distribution, measures of central tendency, measures of variability, laws of probability
- Analyze and interpret data
- Obtaining health information, computing indices (rates and ratio) and making comparisons.

Desirable to Know

- Apply statistical methods in designing of studies
  - Choosing appropriate controls
  - Applying tests of significance (large sampling tests)
  - Use of statistical tables.

VIII. Basic Epidemiology

Must Know

- Epidemiology
  - Definition, concept and role in health and disease
- Use of basic epidemiological tools to make a community diagnosis of the health situation in orders to formulate appropriate intervention measures
- Definition of the terms used in describing disease transmission and control
- Modes of transmission and measures for prevention and control of communicable and noncommunicable diseases
- Principal sources of epidemiological data
- Definition, calculation and interpretation of the measures of frequency of diseases and mortality
- Need and uses of screening tests
- Accuracy and clinical value of diagnostic and screening tests (sensitivity, specificity, predictive values)
- Planning, collecting, analyzing and interpreting data with community participation to reach a community diagnosis
- General principles of epidemiology of communicable and noncommunicable diseases of public health importance and their control
- Awareness of programs for control of noncommunicable diseases
- Planning and investigation of an epidemic of communicable disease in a community setting

- Institution of control measures and evaluation of the effectiveness of these measures.

Desirable to Know

- The derivation of normal values and the criteria for intervention in case of abnormal values
- Applications of computers in epidemiology.

IX. Epidemiology of Specific Diseases Communicable and Noncommunicable Disease

Must Know

- The specific objectives of selected communicable and noncommunicable diseases of public health importance for which National Disease Control/ Eradication Programs have been formulated are described here. For other diseases, the individual teacher would formulate the objectives while drawing the lesson plans. The idea of formulation objectives for a few diseases here is to highlight their importance and emphasize certain learning outcomes.

a. *Communicable diseases*
   - Intestinal infections
     - Poliomyelitis, viral hepatitis, diarrheal disease, cholera, helminthiasis including dracunculiasis
   - Respiratory infections
     - Acute respiratory infections, measles, diphtheria, whooping cough, tuberculosis
   - Vector-borne infections
     - Malaria, filariasis, kala-azar, dengue
   - Surface infections
     - Sexually transmitted diseases, human immunodeficiency virus (HIV) and acquired immunedeficiency syndrome (AIDS), tetanus, leprosy
   - Zoonosis
     - Rabies, Japanese encephalitis, plague, Kyasanur forest disease.

b. *Noncommunicable diseases*
   - Coronary heart disease, hypertension, rheumatic heart disease, cancers, diabetes, blindness and accidents.

- Extent of the problem, epidemiology and natural history of the disease
- Relative public health importance of particular disease in a given area
- Influence of social, cultural and ecological factors on the epidemiology of the disease
- Prevention and control of communicable and noncommunicable diseases by:
  - Diagnosis and treating a case and in doing so demonstrate skills in:
    - Clinical methods
    - Use of essential laboratory techniques
    - Selection of appropriate treatment regimes
    - Follow-up of cases
  - Principles of planning, implementing and evaluating prevention and control measures for the disease at the community level bearing in mind the relative importance of the disease

- Institution of programs for the education of individuals and communities
- Investigating the disease epidemic and the principles of measures of control the disease epidemic
- Awareness of National Disease Control Program.

Desirable to Know

- Level of awareness of causation and prevention of disease amongst individuals and communities
- Control of communicable and noncommunicable diseases by diagnosing and treating a case and in doing so demonstrate skills in:
  - Instituting measures, where necessary, for preventing disabilities/ deformities
  - Rehabilitation of the patient.

X. Demography

Must Know

- Definition of demography and family welfare program
- Stages of the demographic cycle and their impact on the population, concept of demographic gap and population explosion
- Definition, calculation and interpretation of demographic indices like birth rate, death rate, fertility rates
- Reasons for rapid population growth in India and population dynamics
- Need for population control measures and the National Population Policy.

XI. Reproductive and Child Health

Must Know

- Need for specialized services for these groups
- Magnitudes of morbidity and mortality in these groups in the local area and different regions
- Local customs and practices during pregnancy, childbirth and lactation and complementary feeding
- Concepts of reproductive child heath (RCH), components including child survival and safe motherhood, universal immunization program, integrated child development scheme and other existing programs
- Handicapped child
- Organization, implementation and evaluation of reproductive child health program components
- Identify and describe the different family planning methods and their advantages and shortcomings
- Demonstrate skills in motivating a couple for selecting an appropriate family planning method
- Medical Termination of Pregnancy (MTP) Act.

Desirable to Know

- Organization, technical and operational aspects of the National Family Welfare Program and participate in the implementation of the program.

XII. School Health

Must Know

- Objectives of the school health program
- Activities of the programs like:
  - Carrying out periodic medical examination of the children and the teachers
  - Immunization of the children in the school
  - Health education
  - Mid-day meals.

Desirable to Know

- Obtaining participation of the teachers in the school health programs including maintenance of the records, defining healthy practices, early detection of abnormalities, National School Health Programs.

XIII. Urban Health

- Common health problems (medical, social, environmental, economical, psychological) of urban slum dwellers
- Organization of health services for slum dwellers
- Organization of health services in urban areas.

XIV. Health System in India

XV. Health Planning and Management Including Disaster Management

- Awareness regarding important health legislation in India such as Birth and Death Registration Act, Prevention of Food Adulteration (PFA) Act and MTP Act
- Awareness regarding important health legislation in India such as Child Labor Act, Consumer Protection Act, Prenatal Diagnostic Act, Human Organ Transplantation Act, etc.

XVI. International Health

XVII. Geriatrics

PRACTICAL

- Spotters from nutrition, environmental health and entomology, helminths and parasites, occupational health, immunization, maternal child health (MCH) and family planning (FP) devices, etc.
- Problem-solving exercises including epidemiology and biostatistics
- Clinico-social case studies of common communicable diseases, non-communicable conditions and MCH and FP beneficiaries.

UNIVERSITY EXAMINATION PATTERN

Eligibility for Writing the University Examination

The candidate should have at least 35% aggregate in the two of the three internals conducted by the college and should also have minimum 75% attendance in Theory and Practical classes conducted.

Criteria for Passing the University Examination

The candidate should secure minimum 50% in the university theory examination (University theory + Viva voce) and the university practical examinations separately. Internal assessment marks would not be considered for passing criteria, however, they would be added to final marks to determine class of passing.

Distribution of Marks

	Internal Assessment		*University Examination*	
	Maximum marks	*Minimum marks to qualify*	*Maximum marks*	*Minimum marks to pass*
Theory examination	60 marks	21 marks	200 marks	120 marks
Viva voce	—	—	40 marks	
Practical examination	20 marks	07 marks	80 marks	40 marks

Distribution of Marks for University Examination

Theory Examination

It is of 300 marks in total, which consist of:

University Examination	200 marks
University Viva voce	40 marks
Theory Internals	60 marks

Clinical Examination

It is of 100 marks in total, which consists of:

University Practical	80 marks
Practical Internals	20 marks

Theory Examination

There shall be two theory papers each carrying 100 marks. The pattern of questions would be of three types.

2 Long Essay Questions	02 × 10 marks	20 marks
10 Short Essay Questions	10 × 05 marks	50 marks
10 Short Answer Questions	10 × 03 marks	30 marks
	Total	**100 marks**

Distribution of Chapters in Paper I and II for University Examination with Weightage of Marks

Paper I	*Paper II*
1. Evolution of public health and concepts of health 2. Environment and health 3. Health education 4. Nutrition and dietetics 5. Occupational health 6. Medical sociology and community mental health 7. Biostatistics 8. Basic epidemiology	1. Epidemiology of specific diseases communicable and noncommunicable diseases 2. Demography 3. Reproductive and child health, geriatrics 4. School health; urban health 5. Health system in India 6. Health planning and management including disaster management 7. International health

Practical Examination

Practical examination will carry 80 marks.

Ten Spotters	10 marks
Two Problem Solving Exercises	35 marks
One Clinico-social Case Discussion	35 marks

Viva Voce Examination

Viva voce carries 40 marks and encompasses all aspects of syllabus.

Question Bank

	PARK	SYKNT	
CHAPTER 1 **MAN AND MEDICINE: TOWARDS HEALTH FOR ALL**			
Short Answers			
1. List the Indian Systems of Medicine.	2	710	D09(RS2)
2. Add a note on father of medicine.	3	—	D11
3. John snow.	5	—	D10
4. What is the contribution to medical sciences by: (a) Robert Koch, (b) John Snow and (c) James Lind.	5-6	920	D10(RS2)
5. What are the contributions of Louis Pasteur to community medicine?	6	920	J05, J06
6. What has been the contribution of James Lind in community medicine?	6	—	D03
7. Contributions of Edward Jenner (to community medicine).	6	919	J04, D04, D12
8. What is contribution of Ronald Ross to public health?	6	921	J07
9. What is the contribution to medical sciences by: (a) Edward Jenner, (b) Ronald Ross and (c) Louis Pasteur.	6	919	J09
10. Social medicine.	8	3	J08(RS2)
11. What do you mean by "de-professionalization of medicine".	11	—	D13(RS3)
CHAPTER 2 **CONCEPT OF HEALTH AND DISEASE**			
Long Essays			
1. Define health. Describe in detail about indicators of health.	14, 24	6, 9	J15, D16
2. Justify the role of healthy life style in promotion of health. Give two examples of lifestyle factor that promote health and two examples that cause disease. Describe how can you influence lifestyle changes that promote health.	19, 49	8	D02
3. Enumerate the indicators of health and describe physical quality of life index.	24, 17	9, 7	D09

Contd...

Contd...

		PARK	SYKNT	
4.	How will you compare the health situation in two communities? What are the other uses of "indicators of health"?	24	9	J08(RS2)
5.	List the various indicators of health and describe three important indicators which directly assess ill health in the community.	24	9	J01
6.	Enumerate the indicators of health. Describe all the mortality indicators with suitable examples. What are the methods of standardization the mortality rate?	24, 65	9, 218	D08
7.	Describe the concept "natural history of disease" with the help of disease" with the help of a schematic diagram. Mention the levels of prevention and modes of intervention.	41, 47	12, 15	D07(RS2), J10(RS2), D14(RS3)
8.	What do you understand by natural history of disease? Describe citing an examples of a disease, the types of interventions that are possible within its natural history.	41, 49	12, 15	J11
9.	Explain the differences between disease control, elimination and eradication. Describe the activities under the National Pulse Polio Immunization Program.	46, 229	—, 786	J03
10.	Describe the various levels of prevention in relation to natural history of disease and the modes of intervention with examples. Apply each level of prevention to the prevention of coronary heart disease/protein-energy malnutrition in a population.	47, 49	15	D09(RS2), J11(RS2), D12(RS3), D00, J01, J04, D04, D12, J13, J17
11.	You are in-charge of a primary health center. How will you make a community diagnosis of the health situation in order to formulate intervention measures?	56	—	D08(RS2)
Short Essays				
1.	"Tridosha theory".	—	11	D18(RS3)
2.	Four criteria for causality.	—	233	J01
3.	Explain the differences between disease control and eradication.	—	—	D00, J03

Contd...

Contd...

		PARK	SYKNT	
4.	Describe Sullivan's index and how it is calculated?	—	10	D09, J17
5.	Changing concepts in public health.	13	—	D16
6.	Holistic approach in medicine.	14	—	D19(RS3)
7.	Critically discuss strengths and weaknesses of the WHO definition of health.	14	6	J14
8.	Define health. Describe the dimensions of health.	14	6	J12(RS2), D13(RS3)
9.	What are the components of positive health?	16	6	J03
10.	Human development index (HDI)—indicators.	17	7	D09(RS2), J16(RS3), J19(RS3), J14, J17
11.	Determinants of health.	18	8	J16(RS3), D08, J09
12.	"Life style" as etiology of diseases (describe lifestyles affecting our health).	19	8	J16(RS3), D08
13.	How will you measure the health of a community?	24	216	J11
14.	Disability indicators.	26	9	D08(RS2), J12(RS2), D13(RS3), D14(RS3), J17(RS3)
15.	Health-care delivery indicators.	27	10	D16(RS3)
16.	What are the main features of the health team concept?	36	—	D00, D01, J10, D15
17.	What are the various concepts related to causation of disease?	39	11	J09
18.	Describe the epidemiological triad giving suitable examples.	39	11	J01, J07, J12
19.	Describe multifactorial causation of disease with example.	40	11	J06
20.	What is web of causation? Explain with a suitable example.	41	11	D13(RS3)
21.	Natural history of a disease and its stages.	41	12	D08(RS2), J16(RS3), D05, D12

Contd...

Contd...

	PARK	SYKNT	
22. Explain the risk factors in disease.	44	13	D06
23. Iceberg phenomenon of diseases—meaning and application, with suitable examples.	46	14	J10(RS2), D11(RS2), D12(RS3), J15
24. Sentinel surveillance.	47	238	J12(RS2)
25. Levels of prevention. Explain with examples.	47	15	D01, D02, J15
26. Primordial prevention. Explain with suitable examples.	48	15	J16(RS3), D08
27. Describe the health promotional measures.	49	15	D06
28. Explain "specific protection" as an intervention in preventing a disease.	50	15	D13(RS3)
29. Describe the concept of disability with an example.	50	17	J09(RS2)
30. Rehabilitation—types and explain with suitable examples.	51	17	D19(RS3), D12
31. Community diagnosis.	56	4	J09
Short Answers			
1. Sullivan's index.	—	10	D11(RS2)
2. Distinguish between disease elimination and eradication.	—	—	J08
3. Define health.	14	6	D00, J03
4. List the dimensions of health.	14	6	D07
5. What is physical quality of life index (PQLI)?	17	7	D07(RS2), J11(RS2), D12(RS3), D13(RS3), D14(RS3), D17(RS3), D19(RS3), J02, J05, J08, J09, D15, D16
6. What is human development index?	17	7	J10(RS2), J13(RS3), D14(RS3), J17(RS3), J04, D04, J10

Contd...

Contd...

	PARK	SYKNT	
7. What is meant by spectrum of health?	18	7	D07
8. Write about determinants of health.	18	8	D03
9. Lifestyle and health.	19	8	D16
10. What is disability-adjusted life year (DALY's)?	26	10	J10, D13
11. Mention 'health-care delivery' indicators.	27	10	J14
12. What is health team?	36	—	J02
13. Germ theory of disease.	39	11	J12(RS2)
14. What is epidemiological triad?	39	11	D10(RS2), D14(RS3), D02, J10
15. What is web of causation of disease?	41	11	D07
16. Iceberg phenomenon of disease.	46	14	J17
17. Definitions of control, elimination and eradication.	46	236	J09(RS2), D06, J17
18. What is the main aim of disease eradication?	46	236	J01
19. Sentinel surveillance.	47	238	D10(RS2), D19(RS3), D14
20. Describe primordial prevention with examples.	48	15	J05, J14
21. Describe primary prevention with example.	48	15	J04, D03
22. Describe tertiary prevention with example.	48	17	D04
23. Modes of intervention.	49	15	J12(RS2)
24. Health promotion and specific protection.	49	15	J19(RS3)
25. Describe specific protection with example.	50	15	J06, D14
26. Disability limitation.	50	17	J10, D12(RS3)
27. Types of rehabilitation (three examples of rehabilitative measures).	51	17	J15
28. Vocational rehabilitation.	51	17	J19(RS3)

Contd...

Contd...

	PARK	SYKNT	
29. What is community diagnosis?	56	4	J03
30. International classification of diseases.	56	—	J17
CHAPTER 3 PRINCIPLES OF EPIDEMIOLOGIC METHODS			
Long Essays			
1. Define epidemiology and discuss the objective of a descriptive study.	60, 71	215, 221	D09
2. Define epidemiology. What are the types of epidemiological studies designed to explore disease etiology? Discuss in detail 'framework' and 'steps' in conducting the cohort study. Mention the merits and demerits of cohort study.	60, 83, 87	215, 226, 229	J14
3. Define epidemiology. Describe the uses of epidemiology.	60, 99	215, 234	J07
4. Classify epidemiological studies. Describe time, place and person distribution with respect to descriptive studies.	70, 72	221	J15(RS3)
5. Define epidemiology. Classify epidemiological study designs. Write in detail about the steps involved in a cohort study. Write about the advantages and disadvantages of cohort study.	60, 70, 87	215, 226, 229	J17(RS3), D15
6. Explain the term "time distribution of disease". List and briefly explain the types of temporal variation of disease.	72	221	J03
7. Types of epidemics and epidemic curve.	72	222	D16(RS3)
8. Define epidemiology. Classify epidemiologic methods. What is case control study? Write the basic stages (framework for analysis) with suitable examples and mention the advantages and limitations of study.	60, 70, 79	215, 224	J14(RS3), J18(RS3), D13, D06, J17
9. Define cohort. Describe in brief about cohort studies with examples and write a note on its advantages and disadvantages.	83	226	D16(RS3), D19(RS3)
10. Describe the main differences between case-control and control studies.	87	230	J06

Contd...

Contd...

	PARK	SYKNT	
11. What is a randomized controlled trial? Enumerate the different types of randomized controlled trials (RCT). Outline the steps involved in conducting a RCT. Add a note on "blinding".	89	230	J13(RS3), D14(RS3), D15(RS3)
12. Define the terms endemic, epidemic and pandemic. Outline the objectives and steps involved in the investigation of an epidemic.	101, 143	236, 243	J19(RS3), J04, D04, D14
13. Define epidemiology. What is chain of infection? What are the various modes of disease transmission? Describe briefly various measures of prevention and control of communicable diseases against each of the links in disease transmission.	60, 102	215, 239, 244	J09(RS2), J16(RS3), D18(RS3)
14. Who is carrier of infection? What are the types of carriers, give appropriate examples? Write control measures for each of these.	103	239, 244	J12
15. What are the host defence mechanisms? Describe briefly about the various components of the host defence mechanisms.	108	—	J11(RS2)
16. What is cold chain? Describe the cold chain equipments. Mention the factors that determine the effective functioning of cold chain.	117	258	J10, D12
17. Write in detail about "adverse events following immunization (AEFI)" and the precautions to be taken.	122	248	D16(RS3)
18. Discuss in detail about the various agents used for disinfection	140	268	D10(RS2)
19. Explain the steps in "investigation of an epidemic" with suitable examples.	143	243	D15(RS3)
Short Essays			
1. Ecological studies.	—	—	D14(RS3)
2. What is the difference between relative and attributable risk?	—	229	J01
3. Explain differences between an epidemic sporadic endemic and pandemic. Give suitable examples.	—	—	D02

Contd...

Contd...

		PARK	SYKNT	
4.	Differentiate between a carrier and reservoir of infection.	—	—	J05
5.	Differentiate between incubation period and the period of communicability.	—	—	J04, D04
6.	What is the difference between generation time and Incubation period.	—	—	J11(RS2)
7.	Illustrate the elements of cold chain.	—	259	D06
8.	International quarantine.	—	—	J05
9.	Primary immunization.	—	—	J15(RS3)
10.	Define epidemiology. Classify epidemiological study designs.	60	215	D12
11.	Four aims of epidemiology.	61	215	D00
12.	Difference between epidemiology and clinical medicine.	61	—	J12(RS2)
13.	Tools of measurement in epidemiology.	63	215	D15(RS3)
14.	Define rate, ratio and proportion using appropriate examples.	63	215	D17(RS3)
15.	Mortality rates and ratios.	65	218	D07(RS2)
16.	Survival rate.	66	219	D16(RS3)
17.	Morbidity indicators of health.	68	216	D09(RS2), D18(RS3)
18.	Relationship between prevalence and incidence (prevalence vs incidence).	69	217	J14(RS3), J16(RS3), J19(RS3
19.	Describe the different types of epidemics with examples.	72	221	J05, J13
20.	Epidemic curve.	72	222	J10(RS2), D12(RS3)
21.	Explain 'common source epidemics' with examples.	72	221	D14
22.	Propagated epidemic.	73	222	J09(RS2)
23.	What are secular trends? How are they useful to the doctors?	74	222	J11(RS2)
24.	Geographic distribution of diseases and its relevance in epidemiology.	74	222	D08
25.	What are cross-sectional studies? Mention the advantages and limitations of this type of study design.	77	224	J13(RS3)

Contd...

Contd...

	PARK	SYKNT	
26. Explain case control study. Add a note on Odd's ratio.	79	225	D12
27. Discuss the types of bias (in case control study).	81	226	D11(RS2), D12(RS3), J14(RS3), D18(RS3)
28. Write the advantages and disadvantages of case control study.	82	—	D07(RS2), J16(RS3), D03
29. Cohort study—steps, risk measurements.	83	226	D08(RS2), D05
30. Relative risk and attributable risk.	86	228	J18(RS3), D16
31. Attributable risk and population attributable risk.	86	229	D17(RS3)
32. Explain the difference between a case control study and a cohort study.	87	230	J10(RS2), D01, D02, D07, J13
33. Write the steps involved in a randomized controlled trial.	89	230	D09(RS2), D13(RS3), D16
34. Write the uses of epidemiology.	99	234	J12(RS2), D03, J08, D11, J15
35. Cross-over type of study design.	91	231	D07(RS2)
36. What do you understand by cessation experiments?	93	—	J10
37. Different types of association.	95	233	D17(RS3)
38. What is spurious association? How do you prevent it during research studies?	95	234	J11(RS2)
39. Carrier state in disease—salient features, classification with examples.	103	239	J08(RS2), D08(RS2), J09(RS2), D11(RS2), J13(RS3), J14(RS3), J04, D04, J06, D13
40. Write the various modes of disease transmission with examples and control measures based on each.	104	240	D17(RS3), D03, J12

Contd...

Contd...

	PARK	SYKNT	
41. Modes of direct transmission of diseases.	105	240	J15
42. Discuss the various modes of indirect transmission.	105	240	J13
43. Describe the types of transmission of arthropod-borne disease.	106	241	J06
44. Write a short note on biological transmission of arthropod-borne disease.	106	241	J12(RS2), J05, D08, D15
45. What is meant by active immunity?	109	—	D07
46. Primary response.	109	—	D10
47. Herd immunity and its importance.	110	—	J12(RS2), J02, J15
48. Live vaccines.	111	246	J14(RS3)
49. Write the role of immunoglobulins in disease prevention.	114	247	D03
50. Cold chain.	117	258	D15(RS3), J17
51. Cold chain equipment (present in PHC).	118	259	D07(RS2), J15(RS3), J17(RS3), D14
52. Concepts of control.	130	244	J18(RS3)
53. Methods for control of "reservoir of infection".	131	244	J08(RS2), J12
54. Quarantine.	132	245	D16(RS3)
55. Describe the national immunization schedule.	134	250	J18(RS3), J07, J17
56. Immunization for school aged children.	135	251	J03
57. Describe the term surveillance with example.	138	236	D06
58. Emporiatrics (health advice to travelers).	138	274	D18(RS3), D15
59. Types of disinfection.	139	268	D15
60. What is concurrent disinfection? Give examples.	139	268	D09
61. Methods for disinfection for control of communicable diseases.	139	267	J08(RS2)

Contd...

Contd...

	PARK	SYKNT	
Short Answers			
1. What is the difference between secular trend/cyclic tread?	—	—	D03
2. What is geographical mapping of a disease?	—	223	D02
3. Disease outbreak with suitable examples.	—	—	J19(RS3)
4. Difference between and epidemic and outbreak.	—	—	J11(RS2)
5. Differentiate between endemic and epidemic.	—	—	D10(RS2), J09
6. International quarantine.	—	—	D07(RS2), D08(RS2)
7. Difference between quarantine and isolation.	—	—	J15(RS3), J05
8. Mode of action of hand-wash gels.	—	—	J11(RS2)
9. Aims of epidemiology.	61	215	D11(RS2), J14(RS3)
10. Tools of measurement of disease magnitude.	63	215	D07(RS2)
11. What is international death certificate?	64	—	J08
12. Mortality indicators.	65	218	D13
13. Crude death rate.	65	218	D08(RS2)
14. Write briefly on case fatality rate.	66	219	D10(RS2)
15. Direct standardization.	66	220	D16
16. Standardized death rate.	66	220	D09(RS2)
17. List the morbidity indicators.	68	216	J08
18. Write the formula for calculating "incidence rate".	68	216	J07
19. Incidence and prevalence of a disease.	68	216	D13, J15
20. What are the uses of incidence?	69	216	J06
21. Relationship between incidence and prevalence (difference).	69	217	D07(RS2), D03, J10
22. Mention the procedures in descriptive studies.	71	221	J06
23. What are the different types of epidemics?	72	221	D09(RS2), J18(RS3), D07

Contd...

Contd...

	PARK	SYKNT	
24. Epidemic curve.	72	222	D16
25. Write about common source epidemic.	72	221	J08
26. Secular trend in a disease.	74	222	D10
27. Migration studies.	75	—	J10(RS2)
28. Selection criteria and sources of cases in case-control study.	79	224	D11
29. Confounders in a case control study.	79	225	D09, J15
30. Matching.	80	225	D18(RS3)
31. Odds ratio.	81	225	J12(RS2), D13(RS3), J14(RS3), J16(RS3), D15
32. What is bias in epidemiological studies (case control study).	81	226	J01, J09, J10
33. List the types of cohort studies.	84	226	J01
34. Relative risk—define, calculations.	86	228	J11(RS2), D11(RS2), D15(RS3), J05, D07, D13, J15
35. Attributable risk—calculations.	86	229	J10(RS2), D12(RS3), J04, D04, D12
36. Population attributable risk—formula and significance.	86	229	J17
37. Advantages of cohort studies.	87	229	J04, D04, D08
38. Problems in a cohort study.	87	229	J12
39. Advantages and limitations of animal experiments.	89	—	D07(RS2)
40. Write the steps of randomized control trial.	89	230	D03
41. Blinding—define, types.	91	231	J08, J13
42. What is blinding in randomized controlled trials?	91	231	D12(RS3)
43. Spurious association.	95	234	J09(RS2)

Contd...

Contd...

	PARK	SYKNT	
44. Biological plausibility.	98	233	J19(RS3)
45. Enumerate the uses of epidemiology.	99	234	D01
46. Epidemic.	101	236	J16(RS3), D17(RS3)
47. Sporadic diseases.	101	236	J11(RS2)
48. What is pandemic?	101	236	J02
49. Exotic diseases with examples.	101	236	J09(RS2)
50. Epizootic and enzootic.	102	236	J01
51. Define source and reservoir. Give examples.	102	239	J15
52. Disease carriers and types.	103	239	D19(RS3), J02, D08, D14
53. Diseases transmitted by fomites.	106	241	D09
54. Write the criteria for successful parasitism.	107	241	D12
55. Explain dead end infection with examples.	107	241	J06
56. Incubation period—usefulness.	107	241	D00, D01, D08, D12
57. What is serial interval?	108	242	J02
58. Secondary attack rate and its calculations.	108	242	J15(RS3), J13, D13, D14, D15
59. Herd immunity.	110	—	D17(RS3), J14, D16
60. List the vaccine preventable diseases.	111	—	J09
61. Enumerate the live vaccines.	111	246	J03
62. Killed vaccines.	112	246	D16(RS3)
63. Toxoids.	113	246	D15(RS3)
64. Define cold chain and reverse cold chain.	117	258	J19(RS3)
65. Cold chain system.	117	258	D01, D06, J08
66. What is vaccine vial monitor (VVM)?	121	351	J13(RS3), D18(RS3), D02, J02, J17

Contd...

Contd...

	PARK	SYKNT	
67. Hazards of immunization (adverse events following immunization).	122	248	D07(RS2)
68. Quarantine.	132	245	D11(RS2), D18(RS3), D15
69. National immunization schedule (for under-5).	134	250	D07(RS2), J16(RS3)
70. Emporiatrics and its components.	138	274	D02
71. Disinfection—define, properties of an ideal disinfectant.	139	267	D19(RS3), D10
72. Methods of disinfection.	143	272	D16
73. Methods of disinfection of sputum.	143	272	D08
74. Disinfection of air.	143	272	D15(RS3)
75. Epidemiological case sheet for investigation of an epidemic.	143	243	J08(RS2)
CHAPTER 4			
SCREENING FOR DISEASE			
Long Essays			
1. Define "screening" list and briefly describe the criteria for a good screening test. List and briefly describe the features of a disease which make it suitable for screening.	148	264	D10(RS2)
2. Define the term screening for disease. Describe screening for diseases in terms of definition, types, uses, criteria for selection for disease and selection for screening test.	148	264	D01, D08
Short Essays			
1. Screening and diagnostic test—difference.	148	265	J15(RS3), J16(RS3), J11
2. Concept of "lead time".	148	267	J09(RS2)
3. Health screening—define, types, uses.	148	264	D11(RS2), D15(RS3), J17(RS3), J19(RS3), D19(RS3), J13, J14, J15, D15

Contd...

Contd...

		PARK	SYKNT	
4.	Qualities of a good screening test.	150	265	D08(RS2)
5.	Validity of a screening test.	151	266	D08, J09
6.	Sensitivity and specificity of a screening test.	152	266	J08(RS2), J14(RS3), D13, J17
7.	Implications of false positive and false-negative results in clinical practice.	153	—	D17(RS3)

Short Answers

1.	Sensitivity of a diagnostic test.	—	—	D15
2.	Differences between a screening and a diagnostic test.	148	265	D13
3.	What is lead time in screening disease?	148	267	J18(RS3), D01
4.	What are the uses of screening?	149	265	D12(RS3), D12, D16
5.	Types of screening.	150	265	J17
6.	Name any four criteria for a disease to be chosen for screening.	150	265	D13(RS3)
7.	Sensitivity and specificity	152	266	J03
8.	Write the formulae for calculation of sensitivity and specificity.	152	266	J11(RS2)
9.	Predictive value of a screening test.	153	266	J13(RS3)
10.	Give some examples of screening tests.	155	265	D07(RS2)

CHAPTER 5 EPIDEMIOLOGY OF COMMUNICABLE DISEASES

A. RESPIRATORY INFECTIONS

Long Essays

1.	Describe epidemiology, clinical features, complications and prevention and control of measles. Add a note on measles vaccination.	160	283, 285	D10(RS2), J12(RS2), J15(RS3), J17(RS3), D16
2.	How will you investigate an outbreak of meningococcal meningitis in a school hostel? Describe the control and preventive methods to be adopted.	179	313	D10

Contd...

Contd...

	PARK	SYKNT	
3. Describe the problem of tuberculosis in India. Enumerate important epidemiological indices to measure the problems of tuberculosis. Describe the natural history (epidemiology) of tuberculosis and its diagnosis and current strategy in the prevention and control of tuberculosis (drugs regimens) (RNTCP).	189, 191, 193	314, 315, 317	D09(RS2), D16(RS3), J09
4. Describe in detail about directly observed treatment short course (DOTS) chemotherapy in tuberculosis and its 'components'? Describe the 'revised' strategy for the management of patient under DOTS.	201, 457	796, 804	D15(RS3), D15
Short Essays			
1. Describe the Schick test.	—	308	J05
2. Define tuberculosis control in the community. Name at least two countries that have controlled tuberculosis. How could they do it.	—		J11(RS2)
3. WHO strategy for elimination of measles.	160	288	D13(RS3)
4. Measles—natural history, complications, prevention and control.	160	283	D16(RS3), J18(RS3), D07, J13
5. Describe the Koplik's spot.	161	284	J04
6. Measles vaccine.	161	285	D11(RS2)
7. Congenital rubella—assess probability of occurrence, prevention	164	290	J11(RS2), D15(RS3)
8. Discuss the epidemiological features of mumps.	165	291	D12
9. Pandemic influenza A—vaccine and treatment.	169	295	J14(RS3)
10. Pentavalent vaccine.	175	309	D15(RS3), D16(RS3)
11. Write the names of five bacterial agents that can cause acute respiratory infections (ARI) among children. What is the dose schedule of cotrimoxazole for the treatment of pneumonia among children below 5 years of age, as per the ARI control program.	181, 184	280, 282	J11(RS2)

Contd...

Contd...

	PARK	SYKNT	
12. How children suffering from ARI are classified? Write indications of referrals.	182	282	D11
13. Epidemiological indices in tuberculosis.	191	315	J16(RS3)
14. Collection of sputum sample in tuberculosis.	195	—	J14(RS3)
15. Tuberculin test.	197	317	D15(RS3)
16. DOTS therapy in tuberculosis—strategy, advantages.	201	797	D05, J06
17. Write briefly on antitubercular treatment as per RNTCP guidelines.	203	812	D12
18. Give an account of BCG vaccination.	213	320	D10
19. Stop TB Strategy.	219	821	J15(RS3)
Short Answers			
1. Epidemiological basis for eradication of smallpox.	—	277	D12(RS3)
2. What are the cardinal features of pulmonary tuberculosis?	—	—	J06
3. What are Koplik's spots?	161	284	J10, D12
4. Describe rash in measles.	161	284	D11(RS2)
5. List three complications of measles.	161	284	J17
6. Prevention of measles.	161	285	J10(RS2)
7. Measles vaccine (complications).	161	285	D14(RS3), J17(RS3), J19(RS3), J14
8. Write control measures for measles.	162	285	D05
9. Congenital rubella syndrome.	164	290	D12(RS3), D14(RS3), D17(RS3), D18(RS3), J19(RS3), D13
10. Measles rubella vaccine.	164	286	J18(RS3), D19(RS2)
11. What is antigenic shift and antigenic drift?	167	293	J03
12. Prevention of influenza.	168	299	D06, D12
13. Influenza vaccine.	168	299	J10(RS2)

Contd...

Contd...

	PARK	SYKNT	
14. Influenza A (H1N1).	169	295	D17(RS3)
15. DPT—common side effects.	175	309	J11(RS2)
16. Pentavalent vaccine.	175	309	J18(RS3)
17. Vaccine for meningococcal meningitis.	179	313	J09(RS2)
18. Severe acute respiratory syndrome (SARS)—preventive measures.	187	321	J16(RS3), D10
19. Define new case, relapse, failure with reference to tuberculosis.	192	804	D10(RS2)
20. What do you understand by the term treatment completed in tuberculosis?	192	804	D09
21. Mantoux test.	198	317	J11(RS2), D06
22. What is supervised treatment?	201	796	J03
23. Directly observed treatment short course chemotherapy—strategy, components.	201	796	J08(RS2), J13(RS3), J02, J07
24. BCG vaccine.	213	320	D05
25. End TB strategy.	219	821	D18(RS3)

B. INTESTINAL INFECTIONS

Long Essays

1. Describe in detail the strategies for polio eradication in India.	228	786	J14(RS3)
2. Discuss polio eradication in the light of epidemiological factors influencing poliomyelitis.	228	351	J08(RS2)
3. What is the rationale behind pulse polio immunization? List the main activities under National Pulse Polio Immunization campaign in India.	228	786	D02, D04
4. Enumerate the diseases transmitted by feco-oral route. Describe in brief the strategy for the control of hepatitis A.	232	340	J05
5. Discuss the epidemiology, clinical course and prevention of hepatitis B infection.	233	341	D14(RS3), J13
6. What are the epidemiological factors contributing to acute diarrheal diseases? Discuss briefly about its prevention and control measures.	245	329, 333	D13(RS3)

Contd...

Contd...

		PARK	SYKNT	
7.	What are the causes of acute diarrhea? Describe the signs of severe dehydration. How will you manage a child with signs of severe dehydration?	245, 247	329, 330	J14
8.	What are the steps in the investigations of an outbreak of food poisoning in the school hostel located in your area?	262	176	J01, J11
Short Essays				
1.	Describe the intensified pulse polio program (IPPI).	—	786	J09(RS2), J10(RS2)
2.	Describe the steps of outbreak response immunization, with regards to poliomyelitis.	—	789	J17
3.	Define acute flaccid paralysis.	—	789	D16(RS3)
4.	Describe the differential diagnosis of acute flaccid paralysis.	—	789	J17
5.	Chandler's index and its public health importance.	—	359	D16(RS3), D07
6.	What are the strategies for polio eradication? Add a note on pulse polio immunization.	228	786	J13
7.	What is acute flaccid paralysis surveillance?	223	789	D14(RS3), J02
8.	Oral polio vaccine—dose schedule, advantages.	226	350	D08, J10
9.	Mention the steps involved in eradication of poliomyelitis.	228	786	J12(RS2), J17(RS3)
10.	Pulse polio immunization.	228	786	D06
11.	Hepatitis B—modes of transmission/ prevention (primary) and control.	233	342	D09(RS2), J12(RS2), J15(RS3), J17(RS3), D18(RS3), D15
12.	Hepatitis B vaccine—schedule.	235	343	J14(RS3)
13.	Oral rehydration therapy—indications.	247	331	J14(RS3)
14.	Describe the composition of the low-osmolarity oral rehydration salt.	247	—	J17
15.	Write the guidelines for assessing dehydration following diarrhea.	247	331	J06

Contd...

Contd...

	PARK	SYKNT	
16. 'Carriers' in cholera.	253	336	D14
17. Write briefly about measures to be taken to control a cholera outbreak.	255	337	D14(RS3), J13
18. Typhoid fever—epidemiological features/ prevention and control (of carriers).	258	325	J10(RS2), J07, J13
19. Anti-typhoid vaccine.	260	328	J16(RS3), D12, D14
20. Name three communicable/nutritional diseases caused by toxin in the food with examples.	261	173	D03, J05
21. Steps of investigation of food poisoning in a boy's hostel.	262	176	J15(RS3), D08, D14
22. Differential diagnosis of cholera and food poisoning.	263	337	D09(RS2)
23. Prevention and control of food poisoning.	263	177	J15(RS3)
24. Mention food sanitation measures against food poisoning.	263	177	D10
25. Primary prevention of amoebiasis.	264	355	D09(RS2)
26. Enumerate the soil transmitted helminthes and diseases caused by them.	265	357	D10(RS2)
27. Prevention of hookworm infestation.	267	361	D17(RS3)
Short Answers			
1. Define acute flaccid paralysis.	—	789	D16(RS3)
2. What is the composition of super ORS?	—	322	D03
3. What is Chandler's index?	—	359	J12(RS2), J17(RS3), J15
4. What is provocative poliomyelitis?	225	348	D01, D04
5. Salk polio vaccine.	226	349	J15(RS3)
6. Oral polio vaccine.	226	349	D12(RS3)
7. List the strategies of polio eradication.	228	786	J08, D14
8. Mopping up in polio eradication.	228	788	D17(RS3)
9. Australian antigen.	233	341	J09
10. Hepatitis B vaccine.	235	343	J13
11. Rotavirus.	245	329	J15(RS3)

Contd...

Contd...

	PARK	SYKNT	
12. Diarrheal disease control program.	246	823	J09(RS2)
13. Oral rehydration therapy.	247	331	J08
14. Oral rehydration solution—composition.	247	332	J04, D09
15. Assessment of dehydration.	247	331	D15(RS3), D13
16. Briefly describe the rotavirus vaccine.	250	333	D16
17. Dynamics of typhoid fever transmission.	258	326	D09(RS2), J14(RS3)
18. Botulism.	262	176	J15(RS3) D19(RS2)
19. Bacillus cereus food poisoning.	262	176	D09
20. Treatment of amoebiasis.	265	354	D15(RS3)
21. Hookworm—prevention.	267	361	J15(RS3)
22. Deworming.	268	358	D18(RS3)

C. ARTHROPOD-BORNE INFECTIONS

Long Essays

1. What are the factors responsible for resurgence of malaria?	—	773	D00, D01, D09
2. Describe the epidemiology, clinical features and control measures for dengue in India.	270	394	D05, D13
3. Discuss epidemiology of malaria. Write briefly about its prevention and control.	282	367	J13(RS3), D06
4. What is API? Describe in brief the strategy for the control of malaria under national program.	286, 447	369, 773	D03
5. Describe the epidemiology and prevention and control of lymphatic filariasis.	296	376	J06

Short Essays

1. Differentiate between extrinsic and intrinsic incubation period.	—	242	D05
2. What is the radical treatment for malaria as per NMEP?	—	—	J01, J08, J14

Contd...

Contd...

	PARK	SYKNT	
3. Dengue (hemorrhagic) fever—epidemiological features, WHO classification, prevention and control.	270	394	J12(RS2), J14(RS3), J17(RS3), D19(RS2)
4. Management of dengue hemorrhagic fever (in PHC).	277	396	J11(RS2), J15(RS3)
5. What are major epidemiological types of malaria in India?	281	—	D09(RS2)
6. Tribal malaria.	281	—	D15(RS3)
7. What is extrinsic incubation period? Give one example.	283	242	D03
8. Malarial indices.	286	369	D12(RS3)
9. How do you calculate annual parasite incidence? What is the current API in India.	286	369	J11(RS2)
10. Write about the treatment strategy for malaria control.	287	370	D05
11. Clinical manifestation of filariasis.	297	377	J15
12. Why do we take night blood smears? What is the rationale in mass drug administration.	298	378	J11(RS2)
13. Explain filarial indices.	298	378	D00, D01
14. Mass chemotherapy (mass drug administration) in filariasis control.	299	379	J09(RS2), D12(RS3), J13(RS3), D16(RS3)
Short Answers			
1. What is hypnozoite?	—	368	D03
2. Presumptive treatment of malaria—define/for vivax malaria.	—	—	J04, J10
3. Write the radical treatment for vivax malaria/*Plasmodium falciparum*.	—	—	D03
4. Presumptive versus radical treatment in malaria.	—	—	D07
5. Community participation in malaria control.	—	—	D06
6. Mention three gametocidal drugs in malaria control.	—	—	J11(RS2)

Contd...

Contd...

		PARK	SYKNT	
7.	Dengue shock syndrome—manifestations, management.	274	395	J10(RS2), D15(RS3), J09
8.	Extrinsic incubation period.	283	242	J09
9.	What is the cause of relapse in vivax malaria?	283	368	J05
10.	What is man made malaria?	284	367	D01, D04
11.	Name the parameters of malaria surveillance (measurement of malaria).	286	369	J07, J09
12.	Management of *Plasmodium vivax* malaria.	289	370	J14(RS3)
13.	Write the treatment of falciparum malaria.	289	370	J05
14.	Chemotherapy for cerebral malaria.	291	373	J03
15.	Chemoprophylaxis for malaria.	292	373	J03
16.	Malaria vaccine.	294	375	J15(RS3)
17.	Night blood examination.	298	378	J02, J03
18.	Xenodiagnosis.	298	378	D16(RS3)
19.	Mass drug administration for filariasis	299	379	J12(RS2), J17(RS3)

D. ZOONOSES

Long Essays

1.	Describe the epidemiology of rabies and its prevention and control in India. (Write in short about the schedule of cell culture vaccine in prevention of rabies).	302	440, 443	D08(RS2), J10
2.	Describe the epidemiological determinants, prevention and control measures of plague.	320	384	D12(RS3)

Short Essays

1.	Postexposure prophylaxis in rabies/dog bite (antirabies immunoprophylaxis).	304	443	J13(RS3), D17(RS3), J18(RS3), J19(RS3), J08, J15, J17
2.	Write briefly about various vaccines for rabies.	304	444	D05

Contd...

Contd...

	PARK	SYKNT	
3. Antirabies immunization in class III exposure.	305	445	J03
4. Intradermal rabies vaccination	305	447	J05
5. Write the pre-exposure prophylaxis for rabies.	306	448	J04
6. Measures to prevent entry of yellow fever into India.	309	393	J08(RS2)
7. International vaccination certificate.	309	393	D10
8. Japanese encephalitis—natural history/ specific protection.	312	398	D08(RS2), D13(RS3)
9. Kyasanur forest disease—epidemiological factors, prevention and control measures.	315	403	J07
10. What control measures would you recommend for control of Chikungunya outbreak?	316	402	D07(RS2)
11. Mention the methods in laboratory diagnosis of plague.	322	386	D10
12. List the Rickettsial diseases.	326	405	D07
Short Answers			
1. Advantages of Intradermal rabies vaccine.	—	447	D13(RS3)
2. Anthropozoonoses—give an example.	302	240	D16(RS3)
3. Modes of transmission of rabies.	303	441	D09(RS2)
4. Postexposure prophylaxis of rabies.	304	443	D12(RS3), D13
5. List the vaccines against rabies as post-exposure prophylaxis.	304	444	D07
6. What are the indications for antirabies treatment?	304	444	D08
7. Describe the intradermal schedules of cell culture vaccine for rabies.	305	447	J07
8. Describe the pre-exposure prophylaxis for rabies.	306	448	J06
9. Urban rabies.	307	441	J14(RS3)
10. Vaccination against yellow fever (17D vaccine).	308	393	J01, J03, J09

Contd...

Contd...

	PARK	SYKNT	
11. International certificate of vaccination.	309	393	J14(RS3)
12. Amplify zoonoses with examples.	312	398	J09(RS2)
13. Vectors of Japanese encephalitis.	312	399	J09
14. Kyasanur forest disease—prevention and control (activities for limiting the spread).	315	405	J03
15. What is a blocked flea?	320	385	J12(RS2), J17(RS3), D17(RS3)
16. Write five rickettsial diseases with names of vector.	326	405	D03
E. SURFACE INFECTIONS			
Long Essays			
1. Describe the natural history (epidemiology) of tetanus and outline the strategies adopted for its prevention and control.	339	362	J09(RS2), J07, D08
2. What are the factors responsible for the spread of HIV infection in India? Enumerate the personal protective measures for HIV infection.	359, 379	408, 429	J03
3. Write epidemiology of HIV infection. What are the preventive and control measures taken in India?	373, 379	420, 425	D11
Short Essays			
1. Write about the counseling for a HIV positive individual.	—	826	J05
2. Control of trachoma.	337	494	D15(RS3)
3. Tetanus neonatorum—prevention.	338	365	J13(RS3), D15
4. Describe the lepromin test.	347	453	D03
5. Write about the treatment strategy of leprosy eradication (Multidrug therapy in leprosy).	349	460	D08(RS2), J15(RS3), D06
6. Name the deformities in leprosy. Add note on clawing.	354	463	J06
7. Epidemiology of STD's.	359	408	D16(RS3)

Contd...

Contd...

	PARK	SYKNT	
8. Syndromic management of vaginal discharge.	362	413	D15(RS3)
9. Management of genital ulcers.	364	411	J14(RS3)
10. What are the measures for control of sexually transmitted diseases?	367	409	J12(RS2), J17(RS3)
11. Write about the mother to child transmission of HIV.	375	434	D03
12. Prevention of parent to child transmission.	375	435	D18(RS3)
13. Clinical manifestation of HIV infection.	375	424	J15(RS3)
14. Describe common opportunistic infections in AIDS.	376	424	J17
15. Postexposure prophylaxis for HIV.	382	433	J14
Short Answers			
1. What are candidate vaccines for leprosy?	—	462	D08
2. Enumerate the complications of sexually transmitted diseases.	—	—	D09
3. HAART (Human AIDS antiretroviral therapy).	—	425	J16(RS3)
4. Universal precautions in HIV infection.	—	432	D09, D13
5. Define blanket treatment with suitable example.	337	—	J03
6. Prevention of neonatal tetanus.	341	366	D11(RS2), D14(RS3), J15(RS3)
7. What is morphological index?	347	453	J07
8. Morphological Index and bacterial index in leprosy.	347	453	D13
9. Lepromin test.	347	453	D05
10. Fernandez reaction.	348	454	J11(RS2)
11. What are the case finding methods in leprosy?	349	459	D09
12. Objectives of multidrug therapy in leprosy.	349	460	D16(RS3)
13. Treatment for leprosy.	351	460	J12(RS2), J17(RS3)

Contd...

Contd...

	PARK	SYKNT	
14. Write the drug schedule for multibacillary leprosy.	351	460	D03, J04
15. Write the drug schedule for paucibacillary leprosy.	351	460	J05, D14
16. What are the deformities occurring in the leprosy?	354	463	D09(RS2)
17. Syndromic management of urethral discharge.	361	412	J16(RS3)
18. Write case detection in HIV in India.	367	409	J11
19. Contact tracing in sexually transmitted infections.	367	409	D09
20. List out the various routes of transmission of HIV infection.	374	422	J13
21. Window period.	375	424	D09(RS2), D00, D02, J04
22. Case definition used for diagnosis of AIDS.	376	424	J12(RS2), J17(RS3)
23. Western blot test.	378	—	J14(RS3)
24. Write about postexposure prophylaxis for HIV.	382	433	D08

F. EMERGING AND RE-EMERGING INFECTIOUS DISEASES

Short Essay

1. Ebola fever.	384	869	J16(RS3)

Short Answers

1. List the re-emerging infectious diseases.	386	875	D07, D11
2. Preventive measures in Ebola virus disease (EVD)—disease transmission.	384	870	J17(RS3)
3. Control of Ebola virus disease (EVD).	384	870	D16(RS3)

G. HOSPITAL-ACQUIRED INFECTIONS

Short Answer

1. What are nosocomial infections? Give examples.	387	273	J13(RS3)

Contd...

Contd...

	PARK	SYKNT	
CHAPTER 6 **EPIDEMIOLOGY OF CHRONIC NONCOMMUNICABLE DISEASES AND CONDITIONS**			
Long Essays			
1. Explain the epidemiology (risk factors) and methods of prevention and control of coronary heart disease.	398	472	J18(RS3), D02, D04, J10
2. Describe the natural history of stroke. What measures can be taken at the community level to control it?	408	478	J08(RS2)
3. Classify diabetes mellitus. Describe the epidemiological factors causing the increased prevalence of the disease in India.	421, 423	486	D18(RS3)
4. Write about risk factors (multicausation) and complications of diabetes mellitus. Add a note on control and prevention of diabetes mellitus (in district)/Add a note on self-care in diabetes.	423, 425	487, 490	J10(RS2), D11(RS2), D12
5. What are the causes of obesity in India and how to manage this situation.	427	479	J19(RS3)
6. Define accident. Enumerate the types of accident. Give an account of primary factors associated with accidents/ describe in detail the risk factors and preventive measures for accidents.	436	491	D17(RS3), D19(RS2)
7. Describe the epidemiology of road traffic injury. Describe the prevention and control of accidents in India.	438	491	J16(RS3), D09, J11
Short Essays			
1. Write how you will plan for the prevention of diabetes in primary health center area.	—	—	D06
2. Write how you will plan for the prevention of blindness in a primary health center area.	—	—	D05
3. Domestic accident prevention.	—	492	J14(RS3)
4. How do you measure the burden of coronary heart disease in the community.	397	—	D11(RS2)
5. Risk factors in coronary heart disease (coronary risk factors).	398	472	J15(RS3), J04, J09
6. Role of 'diet' in cardiovascular diseases.	398	473	D14

Contd...

Contd...

		PARK	SYKNT	
7.	Prevention of coronary heart disease.	400	472	D15(RS3)
8.	"Rules of halves" in hypertension.	403	476	D08(RS2), D10(RS2), J14(RS3), D03
9.	What are the risk factors for hypertension? Discuss briefly its preventive measures.	405	476	D12(RS3), J06
10.	Epidemiology of stroke.	408	478	J08
11.	Prevention of rheumatic fever (heart disease).	410	475	D16(RS3), D19(RS2), D16
12.	Describe epidemiological triad with reference to cancer.	414	482	D09
13.	Primordial prevention of cancer.	415	483	D07(RS2)
14.	Warning (danger) signals of cancer with examples.	415	483	D10(RS2)
15.	What is cancer registry? Write it's public health importance	415	—	J12(RS2), J17(RS3), J11
16.	Cancer screening in India.	416	484	J13(RS3), J03, J09
17.	Describe the method of screening for cancer cervix.	416	485	D10
18.	Describe the epidemiological features of oral cancers in India.	417	—	J07
19.	Epidemiological determinants of diabetes mellitus (type 2).	423	487	D14(RS3), D13
20.	What are the methods of screening for diabetes mellitus?	424	489	D00, J01, D02, D04
21.	Prevention of diabetes mellitus.	425	490	D13(RS3)
22.	Body mass index—calculation and interpretation.	428	479	J17
23.	Obesity—epidemiological determinants/ assessment/health hazards/prevention and control.	428	479	J10(RS2), D18(RS3), D19(RS2), J02, J07, J13
24.	Preventable blindness—causes and prevention.	430	493	D09(RS2), J15(RS3), J08, D08, J12, D12, D13

Contd...

Contd...

	PARK	SYKNT	
25. Describe the epidemiology and prevention of accidents.	438	491	J12(RS2), J17(RS3)
26. Primary factors associated with accidents.	438	491	J18(RS3)
27. How can we prevent road accidents?	439	492	D08, J14
28. What are the safety measures for accident prevention?	440	492	D01
29. Enumerate domestic accidents and write preventive measures.	440	492	D11
Short Answers			
1. Life style disorders.	—	468	D06
2. What is accident proneness?	—	492	D02, J12
3. Accidentology.	—	—	J15(RS3)
4. List the gaps in natural history of chronic noncommunicable diseases.	393	—	J06
5. Risk factors for (ischemic) coronary heart disease.	398	472	J09(RS2), D14(RS3), J05, D05
6. What is rule of halves in hypertension?	403	476	J08(RS2), J12(RS2), J13(RS3), J17(RS3), J04, J07, J15
7. What is tracking of blood pressure?	404	476	J11, J13, D13
8. What are the non-modifiable risk factors for hypertension?	405	476	J08
9. Write modifiable risk factors for hypertension.	405	476	D11
10. Secondary prevention of hypertension.	407	477	J10(RS2)
11. Natural history of stroke.	408	478	D08(RS2)
12. Risk factors of stroke.	408	478	J18(RS3)
13. Describe the primary prevention of rheumatic heart disease.	410	475	D07(RS2), J06, J08
14. Secondary prevention of rheumatic heart disease.	410	475	D11(RS2), J18(RS3)
15. State the modified Jone's criteria in acute rheumatic fever.	411	475	J10

Contd...

Contd...

	PARK	SYKNT	
16. Enumerate danger (warning) signals of cancer.	415	483	D15(RS3), D18(RS3), D00, J01, J02, J14
17. Cancer registration (cancer registries and its uses).	415	—	J10(RS2), J11(RS2), D13(RS3), J15(RS3), D08, D12
18. Vaccines for cancer.	—	485	J16(RS3)
19. Methods of cancer screening.	416	484	J15
20. Screening of cancer cervix	416	485	J14(RS3), D14(RS3), D15(RS3), J19(RS3)
21. Screening for breast cancer.	416	—	D12(RS3), D16(RS3), D17(RS3), J08, D09
22. Pre-diabetes mellitus.	—	—	J18(RS3)
23. Clinical classification of diabetes mellitus.	421	486	J15(RS3)
24. 'Risk factors' for diabetes mellitus.	423	487	D15
25. State the WHO recommended diagnostic criteria for diabetes.	424	—	J17
26. What is self-care in diabetes mellitus?	425	490	D00, J02, J14
27. Foot care in a diabetic patient.	425	490	J19(RS3)
28. Body mass index.	428	479	D13(RS3), J14(RS3), D17(RS3)
29. Assessment of obesity.	428	479	J16(RS3)
30. List the hazards of obesity.	429	481	D00
31. What are the dietary principles in prevention and treatment of obesity?	430	481	D10
32. List the causes of (preventable) blindness in India.	431	493	J16(RS3), D01, D03, D04, J17
33. Risk factors for road traffic accidents.	438	491	J09(RS2)

Contd...

Contd...

	PARK	SYKNT	
34. Enumerate human factors in accidents.	438	491	D10(RS2)
35. Accident prevention.	439	492	D05, J13
36. Domestic accidents (causes).	440	492	D08(RS2), J17
37. List three measures to preventive domestic accidents.	441	492	D16
38. State the steps in giving first-aid in burns.	442	—	D16

CHAPTER 7
HEALTH PROGRAMS IN INDIA

Long Essays

1. Enumerate vector-borne diseases of public health importance in india. Mention agents and vectors for the same. Describe activities under National Vector-borne Disease Control Program.	828, 445	98, 770	J19(RS3)
2. Enumerate the national health programs related to communicable diseases. discuss in detail the objectives, strategy and implementation of National Program for Control of Malaria.	447	770, 777	J15
3. Discuss Revised National Tuberculosis Control Program.	457	794	D12(RS3)
4. What is DOTS? Describe the strategy for the treatment under DOTS.	457	796	J04
5. Illustrate the diagnostic algorithm for tuberculosis under RNTCP. Describe the various treatment categories. List the major reasons for development of MDR TB.	202	809, 812	J17
6. National AIDS Control Program—explain in detail.	465	823	J15(RS3)
7. Explain in detail the National Program for Control of Blindness.	473	832	D15(RS3)
8. National Rural Health Mission—objectives and strategies, job responsibilities of ASHA.	485	725	J14(RS3), D13

Contd...

Contd...

		PARK	SYKNT	
9.	What is the difference between family planning and family welfare? Describe the components and strategies under Reproductive and Child Health (RCH) Program. Explain the various services provided to the mothers under this program.	499	853	D08(RS2), D14(RS3)
10.	List all the national health programs for noncommunicable diseases. Discuss the strategy for prevention and control of 'blindness' under the national program.	509, 473	771, 833	D14
Short Essays				
1.	List the ten major national health programs.	—	770	J01, D02, D04
2.	List the health programs for mothers and children.	—	545	J07
3.	Write about modified plan of operation under National Malaria Eradication Program (NMEP).	—	773	D08
4	Name the strategies of tenth five-year plan for leprosy elimination.	—	784	J06
5.	Preventive programs for HIV control under National AIDS Control Organization (NACO).	—	—	D06
6.	Measures for control of Urban malaria.	446	774	J08(RS2)
7.	Write a short note on strategies adopted for malaria control.	448	373	D14(RS3)
8.	Describe the role of annual parasite incidence (API) in malaria control program.	448	369	D05
9.	What is active surveillance for malaria control?	449	772	D02, D04
10.	Describe the National Leprosy Control (eradication) Program.	454	782	J10(RS2), D17(RS3), J09
11.	Revised national tuberculosis Control Program.	457	794	J08
12.	Principles on implementation of DOTS.	458	796	D13

Contd...

Contd...

	PARK	SYKNT	
13. Describe the case finding tool for diagnosis of tuberculosis under RNTCP. Add a note on reasons for the false positivity and false negativity.	458	797	J12(RS2), J17(RS3)
14. Describe the strategies adopted by the National AIDS Control Program.	465	829	J10(RS2)
15. HIV sentinel surveillance.	466	238	J08, D11
16. Integrated counseling and testing centers.	468	825	D15(RS3)
17. Explain the components of parent to child transmission (PTCT) program.	468	435	D05
18. What is blood safety? How do you ensure blood safety? What is the current policy regarding blood donation?	471	823	J11(RS2)
19. Briefly discuss "National Program for Prevention of Blindness"—strategies.	473	832	D07(RS2), D13(RS3)
20. Vision 2020.	474	834	J13(RS3), D15(RS3)
21. Universal immunization program.	475	785	J13
22. Scope of health-care (health-care delivery mechanism) in an urban area (slums).	482	730	D06, D14, D15
23. Write in detail about National Rural Health Mission.	485	725	J12
24. Enumerate the components under reproductive and child health (RCH) program.	488	853	D00, J02
25. Essential obstetric care for ensuring safe motherhood.	490	853	J08(RS2)
26. Write the components of child survival under reproductive and child health program.	489	853	J05
27. Nutritional rehabilitation—principles and practice.	492	—	J11
28. Rashtriya Bal Swasthya Karyakram.	498	720	D19(RS2)
29. Describe the strategy under reproductive and child health program.	500	854	D06
30. National Cancer Control Program.	511	835	J09(RS2)

Contd...

Contd...

	PARK	SYKNT	
31. What are the new schemes initiated under the National Cancer Control Program?	511	836	D10
32. Write salient features of National Mental Health Program.	512	839	D11(RS2), J19(RS3)
33. Integrated disease surveillance project.	513	883	J16(RS3)
34. What is minimum needs programme? Comment.	519	860	D01
Short Answers			
1. Enlist various national health programs implemented for mothers and children in India.	—	545	D11
2. Give the objectives of modified plan of operation for malaria.	—	773	J06
3. Comment on malaria week.	—	—	J01
4. Social marketing in family planning.	—	—	J13
5. Enumerate National Health Programs of Vector-borne Diseases in India.	445	770	J10
6. Role of annual parasite incidence (API) in malaria control program.	448	369	J13
7. DOTS agents.	461	797	J16(RS3)
8. Sentinel surveillance for HIV in India.	466	238	D07(RS2)
9. Voluntary counseling and testing center.	468	825	J08(RS2), D19(RS2), D07
10. Social marketing of condoms.	471	—	J08(RS2)
11. Vision 2020: The right to sight.	474	834	D08(RS2), D18(RS3)
12. Reproductive and child health (RCH)—package/components.	488	853	J15(RS3), D05
13. Essential newborn care.	489	516	D07(RS2)
14. What is first referral unit?	490	854	J02
15. Nutrition rehabilitation center—concept.	492	—	J14(RS3)
16. Enumerate the illnesses managed under Integrated Maternal and Neonatal Childhood Illnesses (IMNCI).	494	894	D15(RS3)
17. Adolescent Reproductive and Sexual Health (ARSH) or SNEHA Clinics.	502	671	D15(RS3)

Contd...

Contd...

	PARK	SYKNT	
18. Contraception and adolescence.	502	671	D18(RS3)
19. Integrated disease surveillance system.	513	883	J08(RS2)
20. Swachh Bharat.	517	72	J19(RS3)

CHAPTER 8 MILLENNIUM DEVELOPMENT GOALS TO SUSTAINABLE DEVELOPMENT GOALS

Long Essay

1. What are the Millennium development goals (MDGs)? Critically analyze India's progress in achieving the goals with respect to maternal and child health.	521	683, 689	D13(RS3)

Short Essays

1. Millennium development goals.	521	683	D08(RS2)
2. How many Millennium development goals are related to the health of the community? What are they? Write about any one of them.	522	689	J11(RS2)

Short Answer

1. Millennium development goals.	521	683	J11

CHAPTER 9 DEMOGRAPHY AND FAMILY PLANNING

Long Essays

1. Define population explosion. What are the demographic trends in India? What measures do you suggest for the control of population explosion?	—	562	J11(RS2)
2. Describe in brief the different stages of demographic cycle. Explain in which stage India's population is and how?	530	552	D03, D11
3. Define couple protection rate and discuss the various contraceptive methods used for family planning.	544, 545	566	J08

Short Essays

1. Factors responsible for population explosion in India.	—	563	D07

Contd...

Contd...

		PARK	SYKNT	
2.	Demographic cycle and its stages.	530	552	D09(RS2), D14(RS3), D16(RS3), D01, J09, J10, D13, J15, D16
3.	Population pyramid and its significance.	533	556	J11
4.	What is sex-ratio? Add a note on PNDT Act.	534	556, 918	J13(RS3)
5.	Age pyramids of developed and developing country (like India).	534	557	J15
6.	Write briefly about effects of urbanization on health (Problems of increase in urban population in India).	535	198	D12(RS3), J19(RS3), D19(RS2), D05
7.	Write about life expectancy.	537	558	D08
8.	Factors influencing fertility in a community/factors responsible for higher fertility in India.	538	560	J08(RS2), J06, D09, D15
9.	List out fertility-related statistics.	539	560	D08(RS2)
10.	Significance of 'family size' and its relationship with net reproduction rate (NRR).	540	558, 561	D14
11.	Net reproduction rate and its importance.	540	561	D07
12.	Health aspects of family planning.	542	565	J18(RS3)
13.	Eligible couple.	543	566	J01, J17
14.	Salient features of the National Population Policy.	544	750	D07(RS2), D17(RS3) J19(RS3)
15.	Enumerate National Demographic Goals to be achieved by 2010.	544	751	D10(RS2), D12
16.	Barrier (spacing) methods of family planning/conventional contraceptives—benefits.	545	567	D10(RS2), D07, J09
17.	Write in brief about male contraceptives.	545	567, 584	D11
18.	Intrauterine device—ideal candidate, advantages, contraindications and side-effects.	548	570	J09(RS2), D17(RS3), D13, D16

Contd...

Contd...

	PARK	SYKNT	
19. Hormonal contraceptives—classify, mode of actions, method of administration, effects, contraindications, adverse effects and complications.	551	573	J12(RS2), D12(RS3), J17(RS3), D09, D15
20. Newer contraceptive pills.	552	581	D08(RS2)
21. Emergency contraception/post-coital contraceptive.	552	576	D11(RS2), D12
22. Medical Termination of Pregnancy Act 1971—indications.	557	579	D07, J10, J12, D12, D16
23. What are the natural family planning methods?	558	580	J10(RS2), D08
24. Describe the evaluation of contraceptive methods based on effectiveness.	561	585	J07, D10
25. Community needs assessment approach.	566	—	J16(RS3)
26. Explain All India Hospital Postpartum Program.	567	859	J03, J07
Short Answers			
1. Demographic gap.	—	552	J08(RS2), D13(RS3), D15(RS3), J03, J09, J10
2. Population explosion.	—	562	D07(RS2), D05, J14
3. Zero growth rate.	—	—	D06
4. What is difference between family planning and family welfare?	—	—	J12
5. Role of interpersonal communication in birth control.	—	—	D05
6. Stages in demographic cycle.	530	552	D05, J13
7. Growth rate—define, present growth rate of India.	532	—	D11
8. What is a population pyramid (age pyramid)?	533	556	D08(RS2), D10(RS2), D18(RS3), J19(RS3), D02

Contd...

Contd...

		PARK	SYKNT	
9.	What is dependency ratio?	535	557	J19(RS3), D19(RS2), D08
10.	Population density.	535	559	D12
11.	Effect of urbanization on health.	535	198	D12(RS3), D12
12.	Life expectancy.	537	558	D09(RS2), D06
13.	Enumerate the causes of high birth rate in India.	538	563	D10
14.	Measures of fertility (fertility indices).	539	560	D05
15.	What is total fertility rate.	540	561	D10(RS2), D16
16.	Net reproductive rate.	540	561	J13(RS3), D16(RS3), J18(RS3), J08, J14
17.	Define family planning.	542	565	J01, D02
18.	Target couples.	544	566	J10
19.	What is couple protection rate?	544	566	D12(RS3), D19(RS2), D16
20.	Classify contraceptive methods.	545	566	J11
21.	Conventional contraceptives/spacing methods of contraception (barrier contraceptives).	545	567	D09(RS2), J03
22.	Describe the advantages and disadvantages of condom.	545	567	J06, D11
23.	Intrauterine contraceptive device—advantages/ideal candidate.	546	570	D08(RS2), D14(RS3), J15
24.	Copper T (mechanism of action).	547	570	D16
25.	Postcoital contraception.	552	576	D14
26.	List the important side effects of oral contraceptive pills.	552	575	D10
27.	Enumerate (non-contraceptive) benefits of oral contraceptives.	553	574	J10, J14
28.	(Absolute) contraindications of oral contraceptive pill.	554	575	D16(RS3), J17(RS3)

Contd...

Contd...

	PARK	SYKNT	
29. What are injectable contraceptives?	554	576	D00
30. Menstrual regulation.	556	578	D08
31. What is menstrual induction?	556	578	D09
32. Medical Termination of Pregnancy Act, 1975—indications.	557	579	D11(RS2)
33. List the natural methods of contraception.	558	580	J12
34. Describe no scalpel vasectomy?	560	582	D01, D04
35. Pearl index.	561	585	D01, D04, J17
36. Community need assessment approach.	566	—	D08(RS2)
37. Incentives under National Family Welfare Program.	566	851	J13(RS3)

CHAPTER 10 PREVENTIVE MEDICINE IN OBSTETRICS, PEDIATRICS AND GERIATRICS

Long Essays

1. What is under-five clinic? What are the activities of under five clinics?	—	533	J02
2. What is "at-risk approach"? List the high-risk pregnancies in antenatal care and describe how you would prevent them.	578	511	D07
3. Describe the various methods of classifying 'low birth weight' babies and discuss the important risk factors and strategies for its prevention in a developing country.	587	519	J15
4. Discuss the various health problems encountered in 'children' in a developing country.	601	—	D14
5. Define maternal mortality rate (MMR). Discuss the 'causes/determinants' for high MMR in India (developing countries). Describe 'preventive' and 'social' measures to control MMR.	610	540	J12(RS2), J17(RS3), J18(RS3), D19(RS2), J01, D03, D12, D15, D16
6. Explain causes for reduction of maternal mortality in India.	615	540	J12

Contd...

Contd...

		PARK	SYKNT	
7.	Enumerate the maternal and child health indicators. Define perinatal mortality rate. Write the causes and measures to reduce perinatal mortality rate in India.	610, 617	540, 542	D11(RS2), J13(RS3), D17(RS3), J05
8.	List and briefly describe the various mortality rates of infancy and childhood. Describe the causes of infant mortality in India, and briefly describe three strategies to reduce infant mortality.	610, 622	540, 543	J17
9.	How many infants are dying in India? Why? Explain the causes. How do you prevent these deaths?	622	543	J11(RS2), J04
10.	Define infant mortality rate. Describe role of under-fives clinics to reduce infant mortality.	622	543, 533	D10(RS2)
11.	What are the common causes of under-five mortality in India? Describe the measures taken to ensure child survival in India.	627	—	D07(RS2)
12.	Enumerate the causes of under-five mortality in India. Describe the various national programmers for protection of preschool children in India.	627	544	J11
13.	Describe in detail importance and objectives of school health services in India. Mention various aspects of school health services which are to be provided.	633	537	D07
14.	Discuss briefly the functions and organizational aspects of Integrated Child Development Services (ICDS) scheme.	647	546	J10(RS2)
15.	Describe the various health problems (common organic, psychiatric and social problems) of the aged. Suggest the remedial measures. How can their health and welfare be promoted?	650	661	J09(RS2), D18(RS3), J06
16.	What are the common problems of the elderly? Write about the social security measure for the elderly in India.	650, 759	661, 207	D16(RS3)
Short Essays				
1.	Breastfeeding vs artificial feeding.	—	—	D14
2.	Under-five clinic—aims and objectives/ main activities and benefits.	—	533	J08(RS2), D09(RS2), J06, D10, J14

Contd...

COMMUNITY MEDICINE

Contd...

		PARK	SYKNT	
3.	What do you understand by the term illegitimate child?	—	—	D09
4.	Primary care services for the aged.	—	662	J08(RS2)
5.	Scope of 'social obstetrics'.	573	—	J15
6.	Discuss in brief the 'mother and child' health problems in India.	574	504	D14
7.	Antenatal care—objectives/components (essential elements).	575	505	D10(RS2), J04, D13
8.	Explain the concept of 'risk factors' and give examples of 'risk approach' to antenatal care (high-risk pregnancy).	578	511	J01, D02, D04, J06, D10, J12, D14, J17
9.	Discuss the specific health protection given to the antenatal cases.	579	509	D12(RS3), D19(RS2)
10.	What is mother craft clinic?	579	511	J10
11.	Postnatal care—components/contents of health education.	582	514	D17(RS3), D18(RS3), D03
12.	Complication in postnatal period.	582	515	J19(RS3)
13.	Discuss the objective and steps of early neonatal care.	584	516	D15
14.	Newborn screening.	587	—	J18(RS3)
15.	How will you identify 'at-risk infants'.	587	518	D08(RS2)
16.	Low birth weight babies—prevention.	589	519	J14(RS3), J07, D13
17.	Define exclusive breastfeeding. Enumerate the benefits of breastfeeding.	591	525	J13
18.	Is it necessary to universally breastfeed the babies? Why?	591	525	J11(RS2)
19.	What is weaning and which weaning foods you would recommend for slum children?	592	525	J12
20.	Baby-friendly hospital initiative (BFHI) and characteristics of baby-friendly hospital.	592	529	J02, J03, D11
21.	Growth monitoring in children and its objectives.	593	531	D07, D11

Contd...

Contd...

	PARK	SYKNT	
22. What is the importance of anthropometric nutritional status indicators in preschool children?	595	531	J01
23. Anthropometric measurements in children (to assess nutrition).	595	178	D09(RS2), D03, J12
24. Describe growth chart (used in India) and write its uses (road to health card).	599	531	J19(RS3), J02, D08, J11
25. Write about various child health problems.	601	—	D08
26. Write about the nutritional problems of under five children in your state.	601	—	D05
27. Indicators of MCH care.	610	540	D09(RS2), J18(RS3)
28. Write the formula for the calculation of maternal mortality rate. What are the problems that kill mothers in India?	610	540	J11(RS2)
29. Maternal mortality rate—causes.	612	540	J09(RS2), J09
30. Define perinatal mortality rate? Enumerate the various causes of perinatal mortality in India. Write briefly the measures taken to reduce the same.	617	542	D12(RS3), D08, J13, J14
31. Infant mortality—causes/Factors affecting.	622	543	D09
32. Integrated management of a sick child.	631	894	J08(RS2)
33. Classification and management of illness in young infant.	631	892	D19(RS2)
34. Write the problems of the school age group. How are they being addressed?	633	537	D06, D09, J15
35. School health program (service)—objectives, brief functions, components (different aspects), organization.	633	537	D13(RS3), D00, D01, J05, D05, J10, D13, D14, D15
36. Screening of school children under school health program.	633	537	D07(RS2)
37. What are the causes of mental handicap?	636	535	J07
38. Primary prevention of disabilities in handicaps.	638	536	D08(RS2)

Contd...

Contd...

	PARK	SYKNT	
39. Juvenile delinquency—causes and preventive measures.	639	536	D12(RS3), J09, J12, D15, D16
40. Street children.	642	549	D15
41. Add a note on Child Labor Act, 1986.	644	—	J10
42. What is child placement?	645	536	D02, D04
43. Child guidance clinic.	645	537	J17(RS3)
44. Juvenile Justice Act.	646	—	D17(RS3)
45. ICDS program/integrated child development services scheme—organization, beneficiaries, package of services (benefits).	647	546	J08(RS2), D18(RS3), J19(RS3), D13
46. What is the 'package of services' provided through ICDS?	647	547	J12, J14
47. Enumerate the beneficiaries and the services under (ICDS) integrated child development scheme.	647	546	D05
48. What are the activities of an Anganwadi center?	647	547	D00
49. Write about the organization and benefits under integrated child development services (ICDS) scheme.	647	548	D06
50. Anganwadi worker (AWW)—functions.	647	548	D08(RS2), D10(RS2), J11
51. Write common health problems (chronic) of geriatric population (aged woman) and measures taken to prevent these in India.	650	661	J13(RS3), D14(RS3), J01, D02, D04, D07, J08, J10, J11
52. Enumerate the psychological problems in elderly.	651	662	D09
53. Write briefly about the health status of elderly in India.	651	661	J13
Short Answers			
1. How do you manage postpartum hemorrhage in a community health care?	—	—	J11(RS2)
2. Write the treatment of reproductive tract infections.	—	—	J05

Contd...

Contd...

		PARK	SYKNT	
3.	Under-five clinic.	—	533	J13(RS3), J19(RS3)
4.	What are home available fluids?	—	331	J01
5.	Justify 'mother and child' being considered as one unit.	572	504	J15
6.	Antenatal care.	575	505	D08(RS2)
7.	What advice is given during antenatal period?	578	508	D11
8.	Preventive measures for anemia in pregnancy.	579	510	D05
9.	Congenital syphilis.	580	—	D19(RS2)
10.	What is rooming in?	581	517	J07
11.	Mention the objectives of postpartum care. What are the complications which may arise during postpartum period?	582	514	D12(RS3)
12.	Mention the complications of 'postpartum' (postnatal) Period.	582	515	J06, D10, J13, D14
13.	Early neonatal care.	584	516	D09(RS2)
14.	Write in brief about screening of newborn infants.	587	—	D11
15.	Cretinism.	587	—	J18(RS3)
16.	Low birth weight—define, causes.	587	519	J02
17.	Kangaroo mother care.	589	521	J19(RS3)
18.	What is exclusive breastfeeding? Enumerate the advantages.	591	525	J12(RS2), J17(RS3), J01, J05
19.	Rational for exclusive breastfeeding.	591	525	J11
20.	Advantages of 'breastfeeding'.	591	525	J15
21.	List the weaning food.	592	525	D00, D02
22.	Criteria for baby-friendly hospitals initiatives (BFHI).	592	529	J09(RS2), D14
23.	Growth chart.	597	531	D09(RS2)
24.	Draw a road to health card.	599	533	D03
25.	Uses of growth chart (road to health card).	600	533	J12(RS2), D12(RS3), D02, J08, J10, D15

Contd...

Contd...

	PARK	SYKNT	
26. Maternal mortality rate.	610	540	D05
27. Cause of maternal mortality.	612	540	J13(RS3)
28. Enumerate the social factors which influence maternal mortality.	613	540	D10
29. Enumerate indicators of child health care.	616	540	D10(RS2)
30. Perinatal mortality rate and its importance.	617	542	J08
31. List the medical causes of neonatal mortality in India.	619	542	J07
32. Infant mortality rate.	622	543	J16(RS3), D06
33. Causes of infant mortality in India.	623	544	D07
34. School health services.	633	537	J05
35. School health program—objectives/ components.	633	537	J08(RS2), J10(RS2), D11(RS2), D14(RS3), D11
36. Health education in schools.	635	539	D17(RS3)
37. Behavioral disorders in a child.	639	—	J04, J11
38. Juvenile delinquency—causes and preventive measures.	639	536	J10(RS2), J12(RS2), J17(RS3), J18(RS3), D01, D03, D04, D06, J12
39. Street children.	642	549	J09(RS2)
40. Child trafficking.	644	—	D19(RS2)
41. Integrated Child Development Services (ICDS).	647	546	J14(RS3)
42. Describes the services under (functions of) ICDS scheme.	647	547	D03, J05
43. Anganwadi worker—criteria for selection/ functions.	648	548	D13(RS3), J17(RS3), J02
44. Health problems of adolescents (girls).	649	670	D08(RS2), D03

Contd...

Contd...

	PARK	SYKNT	
45. Health problems of old age/geriatric population (health-care needs of the elderly)—elderly males/elderly females.	650	661	D07(RS2), J10(RS2), D10(RS2), J19(RS3), J05, D12, D14, J15, D15
46. Life style and healthy aging.	651	662	D19(RS2)

CHAPTER 11
NUTRITION AND HEALTH

Long Essays

	PARK	SYKNT	
1. What are micronutrients? Describe their role in nutrition and discuss the management of diseases due to their deficiency.	666, 672	—	D19(RS3)
2. Describe the manifestation of vitamin A deficiency and discuss the strategy of combating the problems at the national level in India.	672, 697	138, 165	D14
3. What are the sources and functions of Iodine? Enumerate the spectrum of conditions under iodine deficiency disorders. Discuss about the components of iodine deficiency disorders control program.	681, 699	144, 171	J13(RS3)
4. Enumerate the nutritional problems in public health. Describe in detail protein-energy malnutrition with respect to its symptoms and preventive measures.	695	162	D12(RS3)
5. What is protein-energy malnutrition? Describe the Ecology/epidemiology, classification, etiology, signs, symptoms, prevention and control of protein-energy malnutrition.	695	162	D13(RS3), J15(RS3), J06, J14, D16
6. Explain role of diet in various diseases. Add a note on 'diet and cancer'.	702, 704	—	D11
7. Describe the methods of assessment of nutritional status of a community with their merits and demerits.	705	177	J10(RS2), J07, D07, D12, D13

Contd...

Contd...

	PARK	SYKNT	
8. Define anthropometry and its role in classifying nutritional disorders in children and their management.	705	178	D10
9. What are the different methods of conducting diet survey and compare their relative merits and demerits.	706	180	D05
10. Define malnutrition. Describe the causes and clinical features of severe forms of malnutrition. How will you prevent malnutrition in children?	708	162	J12(RS2)
11. Explain the influence of socio-economic and cultural factors on the nutritional status of children in India.	708	632	J03
12. What are the sociocultural factors contributing to PEM in India? What measures Government of India is taking to control malnutrition?	708	632	D08(RS2)
13. Give an account of commonly occurring food toxicants in India and their prevention.	713	173	D06
Short Essays			
1. Supplementary action of proteins.	667	134	D15
2. What are essential fatty acids? Enumerate their functions.	667	135	J03
3. Enumerate the water-soluble vitamins and describe any one in detail.	672, 675	137	D18(RS3)
4. Vitamin A—dietary sources/signs and symptoms of deficiency (xerophthalmia) and preventive measures.	672	137	J02, D12, J13
5. Rickets.	674	139	D10
6. Pellagra.	676	141	J18(RS3)
7. Dietary antioxidants.	683	146	D15(RS3)
8. What are alcoholic beverages? Can they give 'empty calories'? Why?	688	151	J11(RS2)
9. Egg—a reference protein.	691	150	D15(RS3)
10. Balanced diet and its components.	694	152	D15(RS3), D02
11. What is balanced diet? Write briefly about the recommended dietary goals.	694	152	J13(RS3)

Contd...

Contd...

	PARK	SYKNT	
12. Dietary goals (prudent diet).	694	153	D16(RS3), D07
13. The Food Guide Pyramid.	695	—	J14(RS3)
14. National Vitamin A Prophylaxis Programme (prevention of vitamin A deficiency disorders).	698	165	D12(RS3)
15. Iron deficiency anaemia (nutritional anemia) and its prevention (anemia prophylaxis program).	698	166	J08(RS2), D14(RS3), J15(RS3), D16(RS3), J05
16. Spectrum of iodine deficiency disorders and its health hazards and their prevention.	699	171	J09(RS2), D14(RS3), D15(RS3), J17(RS3), D06, D08
17. Lathyrism (define, prevention).	701	173	J17(RS3), D19(RS3), D15
18. What is neurolathyrism? Mention the causes, clinical features and interventions for control of the problem.	701	173	D09(RS2), J13(RS3), D11, J17
19. Principles for a diabetic diet.	703	490	J11
20. Discuss the role of diet (nutritional factors) in the causation of cancer.	704	—	J09, J14
21. Discuss various methods of nutritional assessment of a community.	705	177	J15(RS3), J09
22. Anthropometry.	705	178	J09(RS2)
23. Dietary surveys (assessment of dietary intake)—methods.	706	180	D00, J02, J03, J04, D04, J08, D09
24. Nutritional surveillance.	707	181	D10(RS2)
25. Comparison of (difference between) growth monitoring and nutritional surveillance.	707	182	J09(RS2), J10(RS2), J13(RS3)
26. Discuss causes of malnutrition.	708	162	J12
27. Contribution of cultural, social and ecological factors to PEM in the community.	708	632	D07(RS2)

Contd...

Contd...

	PARK	SYKNT	
28. Discuss "cultural influences" on diet, with examples.	708	—	J15
29. Milk-borne diseases.	711	160	J19(RS3), J09
30. Pasteurization of milk—methods, tests to verify.	711	160	J09(RS2), D09(RS2), D10(RS2), D17(RS3), D18(RS3), D15
31. Minimum standards required for slaughter houses (inspection of slaughter house from hygiene point of view).	712	161	D07, J10
32. How would you educate food handlers regarding handling of food?	713	157	D00, D01
33. Food toxicities—food toxicants and the consequents diseases.	713	173	J19(RS3), J02, D05, D09, D10
34. Food fortification.	715	158	D09(RS2)
35. Define the terms: (a) Food adulteration and (b) Food fortification.	715	158	D08
36. Prevention of Food Adulteration Act 1954.	715	159	D07(RS2), J12(RS2), J01, D13
37. Enumerate the community nutrition programs.	717	771	D19(RS3), J08
38. Mid-day school meal and its benefits.	717	539	J08(RS2), D01
Short Answers			
1. What is 'Hyderabad mixture'?	—	165	D11
2. Classification of PEM (protein-energy malnutrition)—Gomez classification.	—	163	J03
3. Differentiate between supplementation and fortification.	—	—	J05
4. Food supplementation.	—	—	J11
5. Write about supplementary nutrition.	—	548	D08
6. List the essential amino acids.	666	133	D10
7. Importance of 'poly-unsaturated fatty acids' (PUFA) in diet.	667	135	D14

Contd...

Contd...

		PARK	SYKNT	
8.	Name three important sources of dietary fibers.	671	137	J01
9.	List four micronutrient deficiency disorders in India.	672	—	D17(RS3)
10.	Vitamin A deficiency—manifestations (xerophthalmia).	672	138	D16(RS3), D10
11.	Keratomalacia.	673	138	D18(RS3)
12.	Schedule for vitamin A prophylaxis.	673	165	D00, J01, D01, D04, J07
13.	Write in brief about deficiency of thiamine in diet.	675	140	J10
14.	Write briefly about beri-beri.	675	140	J17(RS3)
15.	Which vitamin deficiency can cause psychosis? Why?	676	140	J11(RS2)
16.	What are trace elements in nutrition?	678	143	D02, D10
17.	Name four rich sources of dietary iron.	679	143	D12
18.	Name three important items which promotes absorption of dietary iron.	680	143	J03
19.	Goitrogens.	681	144	J14
20.	Dark green leafy vegetable and nutrients present in them.	685	148	D08(RS2), D06
21.	Characteristics of reference adult Indian woman.	689	151	J16(RS3), D01
22.	Dietary needs of pregnant women.	690	152	D08(RS2)
23.	Reference protein.	691	150	D00
24.	Enumerate the dietary goals recommended by WHO.	694	153	D14(RS3)
25.	Balanced diet.	694	152	J12(RS2), D19(RS3)
26.	Mid-upper arm circumference.	697	179	D08(RS2)
27.	What is the dose of vitamin A solution for a 9-month-old child? Why?	698	165	J11(RS2)
28.	Iodized salt (health benefits).	700	172	J14(RS3), D02
29.	Fluorosis (endemic).	701	145	D18(RS3), J11

Contd...

Contd...

	PARK	SYKNT	
30. Lathyrism.	701	173	J08(RS2), D13
31. Assessment of nutritional status.	705	177	D17(RS3), J14
32. Assessment of dietary intake (diet survey).	706	180	J09(RS2), D16
33. Differentiate between monitoring and surveillance with examples.	707	182	J15(RS3)
34. Milk hygiene.	711	160	J19(RS3)
35. Milk-borne diseases.	711	160	D08
36. What is pasteurization of milk? What are the tests used to check for the efficiency of pasteurization (methylene blue test)?	711	160	J11(RS2), J13(RS3), J14(RS3)
37. Method of pasteurization of milk (HTST method).	711	160	J07, J12
38. Write short notes on aflatoxins.	713	175	D10(RS2)
39. Epidemic dropsy.	714	174	D16(RS3), J13, J15
40. Endemic ascites.	714	175	D12(RS3)
41. What is food fortification?	715	158	D00
42. Food fortification and food enrichment.	715	158	J12(RS2)
43. What is food adulteration? Give examples.	715	158	J10(RS2), D13(RS3), D14(RS3)
44. Food additives.	714	156	D14
45. Name the food standards.	716	159	J06, D07
46. Classify and list national (community) programs in nutrition.	717	771	D10(RS2), J12
47. Balwadi nutrition program.	717	846	D16(RS3)
48. School (mid-day) meal program—principles, composition.	717	539	D10(RS2), D07

CHAPTER 12
SOCIAL SCIENCE AND HEALTH

Long Essays

1. Define family. Explain the types of families. Briefly explain the function of families.	738	630	D01

Contd...

Contd...

		PARK	SYKNT	
2.	Describe in brief the role of family in health and disease.	740	632	J05
3.	Describe social factors influencing the health of people.	742	637	J10
4.	Discuss the role of cultural factors influencing health and disease.	742	632	D18(RS3)
5.	What is social security? Describe the benefits under ESI scheme.	758	207, 205	D09(RS2)
Short Essays				
1.	What is marriage counseling?	—	—	J03
2.	How would you do counseling for a newly married couple for family planning?	—	—	D07(RS2)
3.	Write the classification of socioeconomic status for rural area.	—	636	D03
4.	Common health problems among slum dwellers.	—	638	J15, J17
5.	Describe 'social control mechanisms'.	727	633	J14
6.	Discuss in brief the health problems arising out of 'social and economic development' in a developing country.	728	638	D14
7.	Acculturation—effects, role.	728	630	J03, J06, J10
8.	Role of emotions in health and disease.	731	—	D18(RS3)
9.	Discuss briefly different types of 'learning'.	733	—	D14
10.	Family life cycle.	738	630	J09
11.	Define family. What are the functions of a family?	738	630	J13(RS3), J17(RS3)
12.	Role of family in health and disease.	740	632	D11(RS2), J18(RS3), D00, D06
13.	Social and cultural factors affecting health and diseases.	742	632, 637	D10(RS2), D13(RS3), D07, D13
14.	What is social stratification? Discuss how social class affects health and utilization of health services.	744	634, 637	J15(RS3), J02
15.	Describe the relation between disease and social condition.	747	637	J01, D01

Contd...

Contd...

	PARK	SYKNT	
16. Consumer Protection Act.	750	917	J13
17. Operational research.	752	643	J08
18. Diseases of poverty.	756	637	D08(RS2)
19. Social security.	758	207	J14(RS3), J19(RS3)
Short Answers			
1. What is socialized medicine?	—	—	J06, J12
2. Differentiate the crowd from family.	—	—	D00
3. Modified Prasad's classification.	—	634	D08(RS2)
4. What is poverty line?	—	637	J02, J12
5. Social security available for elderly population.	—	207	D11(RS2)
6. Health problems in urban slum/list six major urban health problems.	—	638	J04, D16
7. Define anthropology.	726	629	D06
8. What are the two aspects of sociology?	726	629	J03
9. Socialization.	727	633	D18(RS3)
10. Social control mechanisms.	727	633	J18(RS3)
11. Acculturation.	728	630	J12(RS2), J13(RS3), D02, D12, D13, D14
12. Social pathology.	729	637	D05, J08
13. Cognitive learning.	733	—	J14
14. Intelligence quotient (IQ).	735	535	D18(RS3), J17
15. Categories of mental retardation.	735	535	J18(RS3)
16. Types of families.	739	630	J13, D15
17. Nuclear family.	739	630	J08(RS2)
18. What are the functions of the family?	740	631	D14(RS3), J01
19. Broken family—define, reasons.	741	630	J10(RS2), J02
20. Problem family.	742	631	D11
21. Cultural factors in health and disease.	742	632	J09

Contd...

Contd...

	PARK	SYKNT	
22. What are the social factors affecting health?	742	637	D12
23. Write about medicosocial worker.	749	643	D12(RS3), J08, D10
24. Social security.	758	207	D17(RS3)

CHAPTER 13
ENVIRONMENT AND HEALTH

Long Essays

1. Define safe water. Enumerate the sources of water. What are the various methods of purification of water on small scale?	766, 776	21, 29	D13(RS3)
2. What are the causes of water pollution? Write in detail about rapid sand filtration method of water purification.	770, 773	25	D15
3. What are the various methods of purification of water and mention clearly about household purification of water.	771, 776	24, 29	J19(RS3)
4. What are the guidelines for drinking water quality—criteria and standards? Describe each of the aspects in brief.	779	—	J08
5. Air pollution—sources, effects and prevention and control.	793	42	J18(RS3), J02
6. Define refuse and discuss the methods of solid waste disposal. Write in brief about controlled tipping.	813	65	J09, D11
7. Enumerate the vector-borne diseases and add a note on "prevention and control".	828	98	J14(RS3)
8. Explain the chemical control of arthropods of public health importance.	828	103	D07(RS2)

Short Essays

1. What should be the thickness of plastic bags should they be permitted? Why?	—	—	J11(RS2)
2. Prevention of Indoor air pollution in India.	—	—	D17(RS3)
3. What is green house effect?	—	43	D19(RS3), J05
4. What is ozone depletion?	—	43	D03

Contd...

Contd...

		PARK	SYKNT	
5.	Measures for safe disposal of sullage (in village).	—	75	D08(RS2), D02
6.	Describe soakage pit with a diagram.	—	75	J02, J07
7.	Describe a sanitary well.	769	23	D09, J13
8.	Enumerate water-borne diseases and preventive measures, for the same.	770	23	D09
9.	Mention 'water-borne' diseases and write about the guidelines for 'bacteriological quality' of drinking water.	770, 780	23, 38	D14
10.	What are the steps of water purification?	771	24	D02
11.	Distinguish between rapid and slow sand filter.	774	27	J07
12.	Chlorination of water—principles.	774	27	J16(RS3), D13
13.	Write in brief about break point chlorination.	775	28	D16(RS3), J10
14.	What is residual chlorine? Explain free residual chlorine with a diagram. Is it necessary to have residual chlorine (role of residual chlorine in drinking water)?	775	28	J11(RS2), J02, J04, D04
15.	What are the various methods used for purification of water on a small (domestic) scale?	776	29	J10(RS2), D12(RS3), D18(RS3), D01, D07
16.	Methods of household disinfection of water.	776	29	D11(RS2)
17.	Write how you will disinfect a well in a village during an epidemic (steps in well chlorination).	777	31	J13(RS3), D05
18.	Surveillance of drinking water quality.	779	—	J16(RS3)
19.	What are bacteriological standards of drinking water for rural community?	780	38	J05, D06
20.	What are the methods for determining the bacteriological quality of water (fecal contamination of drinking water).	786	38	D09(RS2), J04, D04
21.	Write the presumptive coliform test.	786	39	D03, J14
22.	Describe the different methods for removal of hardness of water.	787	35	J15(RS3)
23.	Deflouridation.	787	145	D10

Contd...

Contd...

	PARK	SYKNT	
24. Indices of thermal comfort.	792	40	D07(RS2), D16
25. Thermal comfort zone—define, range of corrected effective temperatures for evaluating comfort zone.	792	42	D11(RS2), D15(RS3), J03, D10
26. Air pollutions—major 'air pollutants', sources and adverse health effects/ prevention and control/monitoring (indices of air pollution).	793	43	J10(RS2), D14(RS3), D05, D12, D14, J15
27. Ventilation—standards of ventilation/ types.	798	44	J12(RS2), J10, D10, J13
28. How ventilation and overcrowding play a role in disease transmission?	798, 812	44, 56	J04, D04
29. Lighting standards.	801	—	D16(RS3)
30. Noise pollution—effects on health (noise-induced hearing loss)/control and prevention.	802	46	D08(RS2), D15(RS3), D02, J04, D04, J05, D06, J10, J12, D12, D16
31. Radiation—hazards (biological effects) and prevention.	804	52	D10(RS2), J18(RS3), J19(RS3), J02, J06, D12
32. Criteria for healthful housing.	810	55	D07(RS2)
33. Write briefly about standards of housing.	811	55	D13
34. Housing standards for rural areas.	811	56	D08(RS2), J11
35. Overcrowding and its effect.	812	56	D13(RS3), D16
36. How you will decide the overcrowding in a house?	812	56	J05
37. List the methods of disposal of solid waste.	814	65	J18(RS3), D07, D15
38. Why human fecal matter needs to be treated before disposal?	816	67	J11(RS2)
39. Sanitation barrier.	816	67	D19(RS2), J11, J17
40. Septic tank.	820	70	J14

Contd...

Contd...

	PARK	SYKNT	
41. Oxidation pond.	825	79	D11(RS2), J08
42. Write about the different methods of control of arthropods.	828	102	J13(RS3)
43. Integrated vector control (Culex mosquito).	829	109	J10(RS2), D11(RS2), D13(RS3), D14(RS3), J16(RS3), J01, J14
44. What are various mosquito control measures?	832	102	D10(RS2), J08
45. Explain the antilarval measures in mosquito control.	832	102	D00
46. Write the name of insecticides which are recommended for control of vector of dengue.	832	104	D05
47. Write short notes on residual insecticides.	833	129	D09(RS2)
48. Explain the environmental control of house fly.	834	112	J03
49. Diseases transmitted by soft ticks.	840	122	D16(RS3)
50. Cyclops—control.	842	128	D07(RS2)
51. Give the classification of insecticides.	843	—	D06
52. Rodents—diseases associated/ antirodent measures).	846	—	J06, D07
Short Answers			
1. Nalgonda technique.	—	145	D15(RS3)
2. Fecal borne diseases.	—	—	D08
3. Soakage pit—define, mechanism of action.	—	75	J08(RS2), D11
4. Mosquitoes and immune diseases.	—	—	J19(RS3)
5. List out the differences between mosquito and sand fly.	—	—	D00
6. What are biocides?	—	—	J05
7. Advantage and limitation of insecticides as method of vector control.	—	—	D16(RS3)
8. Safe and wholesome water.	766	21	J06, D07, D12

Contd...

Contd...

		PARK	SYKNT	
9.	Mention the difference between a shallow well and deep well.	769	23	D06
10.	Required standards for a sanitary well.	769	23	J12
11.	Back washing.	774	26	D16(RS3)
12.	Residual chlorine (significance) and its testing in the community.	775	28	D13(RS3), J18(RS3), J11, J14
13.	What is break point chlorination?	775	28	D09(RS2), J12(RS2), D00, D01, J09
14.	Residual chlorination.	775	28	D17(RS3)
15.	Superchlorination of water.	775	28	D06, D09
16.	How do you determine the chlorine in drinking water? Orthotoludine test.	775	29	D09(RS2), J04, D04, D08, D15
17.	Stabilized bleach.	776	27	D11(RS2)
18.	Methods of household purification of water.	776	29	D19(RS3)
19.	How will you determine volume of well water?	777	32	J10
20.	How you will determine the amount of bleaching powder required to disinfect a well in a remote village?	777	32	D03
21.	Double pot method.	778	33	D10
22.	Surveillance of drinking water quality.	785	36	J17
23.	How you will determine the most probable number of coliform organisms in drinking water (presumptive coliform test).	786	39	J01, J05, D09
24.	Horrock's test.	788	32	J10(RS2)
25.	Rain water harvesting.	790	36	D15(RS3)
26.	Indices of thermal comfort.	792	41	D16
27.	Comfort zones.	792	42	D07
28.	Indicators of air pollution.	796	44	J08(RS2), D10(RS2)
29.	Effects of air pollution.	797	43	D07(RS2)
30.	Hazards of noise pollution.	802	46	D01, D15

Contd...

Contd...

	PARK	SYKNT	
31. What is noise-induced hearing loss?	802	46	D00
32. Non-auditory effects of noise on health.	802	46	J11
33. Effects and Prevention of noise pollution.	802	46	J15(RS3)
34. Measures for the control of noise pollution.	803	47	J13(RS3)
35. What is ionizing radiation?	804	51	D02
36. Biological effects of radiation (effects of radiation on health).	804	52	J12(RS2), J14(RS3), J07, J08
37. Effects of atmospheric pressure on health.	806	58	J09(RS2)
38. Health hazards due to exposure to high temperature.	807	61	D05
39. Kata thermometer.	807	64	D15(RS3)
40. Effects of heat stress.	807	62	J18(RS3)
41. What is heat hyperpyrexia?	808	—	J01
42. Global warming.	808	889	D18(RS3)
43. Waste disposal in urban areas.	814	65	J19(RS3)
44. Composting.	815	66	J18(RS3), D19(RS3)
45. What is sanitary barrier?	816	67	J08(RS2), J13(RS3), J05, D14
46. List out four criteria of a sanitary latrine.	817	67	D01
47. Mention two uses of water seal in a water seal latrine.	818	68	J03
48. What are the methods of sewage disposal.	823	76	D10(RS2)
49. Oxidation pond.	825	79	J11, J17
50. Write five vector-borne diseases with names of vector.	828	98	J04
51. What is biological control of vectors?	828	104	J04, D04, J13
52. Integrated vector control measures	829	109	J15(RS3)
53. Aedes mosquitoes and disease.	831	106	D13(RS3)
54. What is Aedes aegypti index?	831	393	J13(RS3), D09
55. Antimosquito measures.	832	102	D15(RS3)

Contd...

Contd...

	PARK	SYKNT	
56. Environmental antilarval measures.	832	102	D08(RS2)
57. Residual insecticides.	833	129	J03, D09
58. Diseases transmitted through house flies.	834	112	D08
59. List out the public health importance of sand fly.	836	113	J01
60. List out the diseases transmitted by lice.	837	119	D01
61. What are flea indices?	839	118	J02, D08, D13
62. Mention tick-borne diseases.	840	122	J11(RS2)
63. Write briefly on itch mite.	841	125	J09
64. Prevention of scabies.	842	126	D19(RS3), J07
65. Discuss the mechanism of action, uses and public health importance of dichlorodiphenyltrichloroethane (DDT).	843	105	J13
66. List the diseases transmitted by rats.	846	—	D07
67. What are rodenticides?	847	—	D07(RS2), D03
68. Enumerate the important zoonatic diseases.	848	240	D10(RS2)

CHAPTER 14
HOSPITAL WASTE MANAGEMENT

Long Essay

1. What are various methods of treatment and disposal technologies for health-care waste?	850	85	D09(RS2)

Short Essays

1. How biomedical waste is categorized? How category No. 3 is disposed off?	—	83	D11
2. What is category No. 3 of biomedical wastes and how it is treated/disposed?	—	83	J07
3. Health hazards of health-care waste.	850	80	J09(RS2)
4. Categories of Biomedical waste in India.	853	83	D17(RS3)
5. Write the different containers and their colors for disposing the hospital wastes.	853	83	J04, D04

Contd...

Contd...

	PARK	SYKNT	
Short Answer			
1. Genotoxic waste.	850	—	D19(RS2)

CHAPTER 15
DISASTER MANAGEMENT

	PARK	SYKNT	
Short Essays			
1. Training in disaster management.	—	—	D06
2. What is a disaster? Enumerate the different types of disasters.	855	877	J19(RS3), D00, D01
3. Disaster cycle.	857	878	D18(RS3), D14
4. 'Aspects' of disaster management.	857	878	D15
5. What are short—term effects of disaster?	856	877	D11
6. List the ten health/medical activities during disaster management/disaster mitigation.	858	879	J01, D02, D04, D11
7. What is disaster preparedness? List six components of disaster preparedness.	859	879	D12(RS3), J13(RS3), J02
8. What are the health and environmental problems due to floods?	860	880	D10
9. Disaster management in floods.	860	881	D17(RS3)
10. Manmade disasters and its preventive measures.	862	878	D19(RS2), D07
11. Disaster management in India.	862	—	J14(RS3)
Short Answers			
1. Disaster—define/types.	855	877	D07, D14
2. Disaster cycle.	857	878	J15(RS3)
3. What is 'triage'. Scope of 'triage' in dealing with emergencies/disaster management.	857	879	J13(RS3), D14(RS3), J16(RS3), D16(RS3), J17(RS3), D09, D13, D15
4. Disaster (earthquake) mitigation in health sector.	858	879	D09(RS2), D11(RS2), D13(RS3), J14

Contd...

Contd...

		PARK	SYKNT	
5.	Disaster preparedness.	859	879	D12
6.	Pre-disaster phase of disaster management.	859	879	J08(RS2)
7.	Man-made disasters.	862	878	J18(RS3)

CHAPTER 16
OCCUPATIONAL HEALTH

Long Essays

1.	Classify occupational diseases. Describe the various measures for the prevention of occupational diseases.	866, 873	188, 201	J16(RS3), D07
2.	Classify occupational diseases. Write in detail about the engineering measures to prevent occupational diseases.	866, 874	188, 201	J15
3.	Define occupational health. List the occupational hazards. Mention the legislative measures to prevent them.	866, 876	187, 204	D10
4.	What is pneumoconiosis? What are the factors that influence causation of pneumoconiosis? Describe the various types of pneumoconiosis and their health effects? What measures are taken to prevent it?	867	189	J12(RS2), D05
5.	Define pneumoconiosis. How is silicosis caused and how is it prevented?	867	189	D00
6.	What are the health hazards of workers in coal mines? What steps you would take to reduce the hazards?	867, 873	191	J08(RS2)
7.	Describe in detail, the various health problems due to industrialization.	871	198	D17(RS3)
8.	What are the laws meant for the protection of industrial workers? Write in detail about Factories Act, 1948.	876	204	D11(RS2)
9.	Explain the differences between social assistance and social insurance. Enumerate the provisions under the Indian Factory Act.	876	208, 204	J02
10.	Write in detail about the benefits available to the employees and employers under the Employees State Insurance (ESI) Act, 1948?	877	205	J13

Contd...

Contd...

	PARK	SYKNT	
Short Essays			
1. How can one prevent the hazards of agricultural occupation in India?	—	197	J09
2. Classify occupational diseases with examples.	866	188	J10(RS2)
3. Pneumoconiosis (name giving occupation where they occur).	867	189	D10(RS2), J15(RS3), J19(RS3), J05, D08, J14
4. Silicosis—epidemiology, manifestation and measures of control.	867	190	D13(RS3), D01, D06
5. Anthracosis.	867	191	D15
6. General measures for control of pneumoconiosis.	868	192	J11
7. Outline causes, clinical features, management and prevention of lead poisoning (plumbism).	868	193	D11(RS2), J15(RS3), J18(RS3), D09, J15, D16
8. Occupational cancers.	869	195	D07(RS2), D10(RS2), J12(RS2), J04, D04, J08, D13
9. Occupational dermatitis.	870	196	J14(RS3)
10. Explain the occupation hazards of agriculture workers.	870	197	J09(RS2), D01, J07
11. Prevention of industrial accidents.	871	198	D17(RS3)
12. What is sickness absenteeism? Enumerate the reasons. Explain the significance of sickness absentism.	871	200	J17(RS3), D09, J10
13. Health problems due to industrialization.	871	198	J10(RS2), D18(RS3)
14. What (medical) measures can be taken to protect the workers health?	873	201	D09(RS2), D14(RS3), J09
15. Pre-employment medical examination.	873	201	D00, J06, D07, D11
16. Explain the advantages of pre-placement and periodic medical examinations in occupational health.	873	201, 203	D02

Contd...

Contd...

	PARK	SYKNT	
17. Explain with examples, periodic medical examination.	874	203	J01, J02, J03
18. Provisions under Factories Act, 1948—health promotion/health safety and welfare provisions.	876	204	J08(RS2), J12
19. Employees State Insurance Act, 1948—benefits to employees (sickness/medical).	877	205	D10(RS2), J11(RS2), D12(RS3), J15(RS3), D19(RS3), D02, J04, D04, J05, J08, J11, D11, D12
Short Answers			
1. Occupational hazards of health-care professionals.	—	—	D17(RS3)
2. Ergonomics.	864	187	D19(RS3), J04, D04, J07, J15, D16
3. Effect of vibration on health.	865	188	J11
4. What is respirable dust?	866	189	D02
5. Define silicosis. How is it diagnosed?	867	190	D17(RS3)
6. Anthracosis.	867	191	D18(RS3)
7. What is bagassosis?	868	192	J10, D14
8. Asbestosis and control.	868	191	D08(RS2), J13(RS3)
9. Dust control measures in coal mines.	868	192	J12
10. Farmer's lung.	868	192	D09, J17
11. Lead poisoning (plumbism).	868	193	D10
12. Occupational cancers—enumerate, causes.	869	195	J10(RS2), D08, J13
13. Cancer in dye industries.	869	195	J11(RS2)
14. Occupational dermatitis—causes and prevention.	870	196	J09, J15
15. Occupational risk to farmers/agricultural workers.	870	197	D11(RS2), D12(RS3), D18(RS3)

Contd...

Contd...

	PARK	SYKNT	
16. Sickness absenteeism—define/ measures for prevention.	871	200	D14(RS3), J06, D11, D12, J14
17. Preplacement examination and its importance.	873	201	J08(RS2), D19(RS3), D15
18. List the engineering measures to prevent occupational diseases.	874	202	J18(RS3)
19. The Factories Act, 1948.	876	204	D09
20. Employees State Insurance Act—benefits (medical/sickness/maternity).	877	205	D09(RS2), J16(RS3), J03

CHAPTER 17
GENETICS AND HEALTH

Short Essays

1. Genetic engineering.	—	—	J18(RS3)
2. Chromosomal abnormalities.	882	657	D07(RS2)
3. Down's syndrome.	883	658	D13(RS3)
4. Write in brief the role of genetic predisposition in common disorders.	886	659	J10
5. DNA recombinant technology.	887	—	D18(RS3), D19(RS2)
6. What is population genetics?	888	657	J02
7. Prevention of genetic disorders (Klinefilter's syndrome).	888	659	D11(RS2), D12(RS3), J09, D11
8. What is eugenics?	888	659	D03, J04
9. Genetic counseling.	889	659	J18(RS3), D00, D01, J07, J14
10. Consanguinous marriage.	889	—	D10

Short Answers

1. Difference between eugenic and euthenics.	—	—	J14(RS3)
2. Enumerate Mendel's laws of inheritance.	883	657	D11(RS2)
3. Down's syndrome.	883	658	D18(RS3)
4. What is Klinefelter syndrome?	883	658	J07

Contd...

Contd...

	PARK	SYKNT	
5. Human genome project.	887	—	D07(RS2)
6. Population genetics.	888	657	D11(RS2)
7. Hardy Weinberg law.	888	—	J13(RS3)
8. Define the terms 'euthenics and 'eugenics'.	888	659	J17
9. Eugenics—application in medicine.	888	659	J04, D04, D05, D06, D10, D14, D15
10. What is euthenics?	889	659	D13(RS3), D19(RS2), J14
11. What is prospective genetic counseling?	889	659	D10

CHAPTER 18
MENTAL HEALTH

Short Essays

	PARK	SYKNT	
1. What are illusions, delusions and hallucinations.	—	—	J11(RS2)
2. What is primary mental health care and how is it implemented.	—	—	J12
3. Write the characteristics of mentally healthy individual.	892	—	J11
4. Warning signals of poor mental health.	893	—	J09(RS2)
5. Common mental health problems.	893	—	J13
6. What are the causes of mental ill health?	894	666	J08
7. Types of mental illness.	893	666	J14(RS3), D18(RS3)
8. Mental health services in India	895	—	D16(RS3)
9. Drug dependence/addiction.	895	674	D07(RS2), D10
10. Socioeconomic effects of smoking.	897	911	J16(RS3)
11. Adverse health effects of smoking.	899	911	D15(RS3), D19(RS3)
12. Factors associated with a high risk for drug abuse.	900	674	J18(RS3)

Contd...

Contd...

	PARK	SYKNT	
13. Role of legislation in reducing alcoholism in the society.	900	677	D17(RS3)
Short Answers			
1. Warning signs of poor mental health.	893	—	D08(RS2), D09(RS2), D10(RS2), D11(RS2), J16(RS3), J11
2. Causes of mental ill health.	894	666	J17
3. Mental health services in India	895	—	J15(RS3)
4. What is comprehensive mental health program?	895	—	J09
5. List the drugs causing dependence.	895	675	J06
6. Passive smoking.	898	676	J14(RS3)
7. Discuss the effects of tobacco use. What are the preventive measures?	899	911	J17(RS3)
8. Measures for prevention of smoking.	900	912	J14(RS3)
9. List the factors associated with a high risk for drug abuse.	900	674	D06, J13
10. Prevention of drug dependence.	900	676	J16(RS3)
11. Recommend solution for the problem of drug abuse in India.	900	676	D17(RS3)
12. Explain de-addiction.	900	676	J02

CHAPTER 19
HEALTH INFORMATION AND BASIC MEDICAL STATISTICS

Long Essay			
1. What is sampling? Explain with suitable examples the different methods of sampling.	912	603	J16(RS3), D02, J05
Short Essays			
1. What is the difference between standard deviation and standard error?	—	—	D07
2. Explain cluster sampling with examples.	—	605	J02, J12
3. Health information system—define, components and uses.	902	—	J13(RS3), D01, J07, D11, J13

Contd...

COMMUNITY MEDICINE

Contd...

		PARK	SYKNT	
4.	Enumerate various sources of health information system in India. Describe any one in detail.	903	588	D09(RS2), J11, D13
5.	What are the different sources of health information? What are the disadvantages of hospital records.	903	588	J11(RS2)
6.	Write briefly on census.	903	552	D02, D04, J08
7.	Write briefly on sample registration system.	904	553	J13
8.	Notification of diseases—list and its merits and demerits.	904	—	D16(RS3), J06, J09, D14
9.	Write merits and dements of hospital records as source of health information.	904	588	J12
10.	Medical record linkage.	905	238	J14(RS3), D16
11.	National Family Health Survey.	906	553	D16
12.	Bar charts	907	590	J17(RS3), D15
13.	What are the measures of central tendency? What are its limitations?	910	596	D10(RS2), D19(RS3), J01, D11
14.	Statistical averages.	910	596	D12
15.	What are the measures of dispersion?	911	597	J16(RS3), D00, D01, J07, J08
16.	Standard deviation.	911	598	D15(RS3), D10
17.	Normal curve and normal distribution—characteristics.	912	600	D14(RS3), D17(RS3), J12, J15
18.	What is sampling? Enumerate the techniques (sampling methods/ techniques).	912	603	J17(RS3), D17(RS3), D09, J11, D15
19.	Simple random sampling.	913	603	J17(RS3)
20.	What is stratified random sampling? Illustrate with an example.	913	604	D13(RS3), J03, J10, D13
21.	Sampling error.	913	606	J17

Contd...

Contd...

	PARK	SYKNT	
22. Describe briefly the various "tests of significance"	913	608	J08(RS2), D11(RS2), J17
23. Chi-square test.	915	613	D16
Short Answers			
1. Quantitative variables, give example of each.	—	589	D05
2. Meaning of the term "inter-quartile range"	—	—	D09(RS2)
3. Contingency table.	—	—	J09(RS2)
4. Law of probability.	—	599	D05
5. Cluster sampling.	—	605	D00
6. What is data? Write types with suitable examples.	902	587	D11
7. Distinguish between data and information.	902	—	D08
8. Write uses of health information system.	902	—	J12
9. Sources of health information.	903	588	D09(RS2), D08
10. Census as source of health information.	903	552	J10(RS2), D11, D13
11. What is vital statistics? Write its sources in India.	903	588	D11
12. Vital events—registration.	903	—	D12(RS3), J14(RS3), D18(RS3)
13. Birth and Death Registration Act of 1969.	903	917	D08(RS2), D16(RS3)
14. What is 'Lay reporting'?	903	—	J14
15. Sample registration system.	904	553	D17(RS3), J15
16. What is dual registration system?	904	—	J12
17. Hospital records—three drawbacks/five uses.	904	588	D00, D01, J02, D04
18. Record linkage.	905	238	J09(RS2), D11(RS2), D15(RS3), J16(RS3), J11

Contd

Contd...

	PARK	SYKNT	
19. Bar diagram (Bar charts) and its uses.	907	590	D08(RS2), J10(RS2), J14(RS3), D15(RS3)
20. Histogram.	908	590	J09(RS2), J01, J12
21. Pie chart.	909	593	D00, D07, J15
22. What is spot map?	—	594	J13(RS3), D01, J07, D12
23. Measures of central tendency.	910	596	D14(RS3), J15(RS3), D03, J06, J12
24. Standard normal curve—properties/ draw.	912	600	D08(RS2), J17(RS3), J18(RS3), D06, J13, J17
25. Sampling methods/types.	913	603	D16(RS3), J19(RS3), J09
26. Stratified random sampling.	913	604	J08(RS2)
27. Sampling errors.	913	606	D09(RS2)
28. Name the tests of significance.	913	608	J18(RS3)
29. Chi-square test.	915	613	D15(RS3), J17(RS3)

CHAPTER 20 COMMUNICATION FOR HEALTH EDUCATION

Long Essays

1. Define health education and describe the various approaches and applications of health education.	920, 926	647	J09
2. What is health education? Discuss the principles of health education giving examples. Write briefly about the communication process. Enumerate the steps in planning for conducting a health educational session in a village.	920, 924, 917	647, 646	D11(RS2), J17(RS3)

Contd...

Contd...

		PARK	SYKNT	
3.	What is health education? Discuss how you will organize a health education session on anemia for village women.	920, 930	647	J12
4.	What are the contents and principles of health education?	923	648	J08
5.	What is concept of information, education and communication? Describe in brief the various methods to deliver it.	926	646, 649	D03
6.	Classify and describe the various methods of health communication. Enlist the advantages and disadvantages of the different methods.	926	649	J09(RS2), D17(RS3)
Short Essays				
1.	Effective methods of communication to youths.	—	—	J08(RS2)
2.	Barriers of health communication and their prevention.	919	647	J10(RS2), J12(RS2), D12(RS3), D13(RS3), J15(RS3), J11
3.	Functions of 'health communication'.	919	—	J14
4.	Define health education. Describe six stages of adoption of new ideas and practices with one example.	920	647	D00, D02
5.	Briefly discuss the various approaches to health education.	921	648	D09(RS2), D14(RS3)
6.	Models of health education.	922	648	D19(RS3)
7.	Enumerate the differences between health education and health propaganda.	922	648	D10(RS2), J06, J07
8.	Principles of health education.	924	648	D08(RS2), J09(RS2), J13(RS3), J13, D13, J17
9.	What is group health education? Write in brief about lectures.	927	650	J01
10.	What is group health discussion? Write in brief about group discussion.	927	650	D16
11.	What is group health education? Write in brief about role play.	928	652	J03
12.	Discuss in brief the various health education methods for mass education.	929	654	D05

Contd...

Contd...

	PARK	SYKNT	
13. 'Mass approach' for health education (mass media).	929	654	D11, J14, D15
Short Answers			
1. What is an effective communication?	—	—	J05
2. Difference between seminar and symposium.	—	—	D05
3. Types of communication.	918	647	J16(RS3), J15
4. Barriers of communication.	919	647	D15(RS3)
5. List the functions of health communication.	919	—	D06
6. Health education and propaganda—difference.	922	648	J13(RS3)
7. Principles of health education.	924	648	D12
8. Different methods of health education.	926	649	J04, D04
9. Write modern methods of communication in medicine.	926	647	J11
10. Audiovisual aids in health education.	926	649	D11(RS2), J02, D09
11. Write advantages of individual approach in health education.	926	650	D11
12. Explain in brief what is a group discussion.	927	650	D12(RS3), J10, J14
13. Panel discussion.	928	651	J10(RS2), J16(RS3), J11, D14
14. What is role play?	928	652	J07
15. Symposium.	928	651	J12(RS2), D14(RS3)
16. Mass media for health education—advantages and disadvantages.	929	654	J14(RS3)
17. Enumerate the uses of Internet in medicine.	929	914	D02

CHAPTER 21
HEALTH PLANNING AND MANAGEMENT

Long Essays			
1. What is meant by National Health Planning? Describe the steps involved in a planning cycle.	931	739, 735	D10

Contd...

Contd...

		PARK	SYKNT	
2.	Describe the various stage of planning cycle.	932	735	D06
3.	Define management. Describe the management methods and techniques.	933	736	J09
Short Essays				
1.	Differentiate between a cost effective and cost benefit study.	—	—	J04
2.	Define objective, target and goal.	931	735	D09
3.	Explain stages of planning cycle with a diagram.	932	735	J08(RS2), D08(RS2), D10(RS2), D13(RS3), D00, J01, J02, J03, D03, D05, J15, J17
4.	Management techniques based on behavioral sciences.	934	—	D11(RS2)
5.	Describe cost benefit analysis.	934	737	D14(RS3), J06, J10
6.	Input-output analysis.	934	—	D16
7.	Network analysis.	935	736	J14
8.	Program evaluation review technique (PERT)—advantages.	935	736	D10(RS2)
9.	Describe salient points of National Health Policy, 2002.	936	748	J10(RS2), D05
10.	Write the recommendations of Bhore committee.	937	739	J19(RS3), J04, J12, D16
11.	Write three recommendations of Mudaliar committee.	937	739	D03
12.	Write the recommendations of Kartar Singh committee.	938	740	J05
13.	Describe the purpose and recommendations of Shrivastav committee.	938	740	J10(RS2), J16(RS3), J18(RS3)
14.	Rural health scheme.	939	—	J08
15.	Enumerate organizational structure of health system in India.	942	743	J15

Contd...

Contd...

	PARK	SYKNT	
16. Central health council and its functions.	943	744	J10, J11
17. Write in brief about role of Gram Sevak in Panchayati Raj.	946	746	D09
18. List out the basic steps involved in evaluation.	946	—	J09(RS2)
Short Answers			
1. Write differences between cost-effective and cost-benefit analysis.	—	—	D11
2. What is pre-planning?	932	—	D13
3. Planning cycle and its steps.	932	735	J07, J09
4. Management by objectives (advantages).	934	—	D07(RS2), J12
5. Enumerate 'quantitative' methods of management.	934	—	D15
6. What is cost benefit and cost effectiveness?	934	737	J01, D02
7. Cost benefit analysis.	934	737	D12, J14
8. Cost effective analysis.	934	737	D13(RS3)
9. Input-output analysis.	934	—	J09(RS2), D10
10. Network analysis.	935	736	J10(RS2), J12(RS2), J17(RS3)
11. Program evaluation review technique.	935	736	D16(RS3), D16
12. Explain through a line diagram what is critical path method.	935	737	J07, J08, D09, D14
13. Planning-programming-budgeting system.	935	—	D11(RS2)
14. Recommendations of Bhore committee.	937	739	D13(RS3)
15. Recommendations of Shrivastav committee, 1975.	938	740	J09(RS2), D12(RS3)
16. Five-year plans.	939	740	J08(RS2)
17. 'Evaluation' of health programme (planning)—components/general steps.	946	—	J11, J15

Contd...

Contd...

	PARK	SYKNT	
CHAPTER 22 **HEALTH CARE OF THE COMMUNITY**			
Long Essays			
1. Define primary health care. List the elements of primary health care. Briefly explain the principles of primary health care.	951	699	D01, D05, J13
2. Define primary health care. What are its components? Describe how primary health care is provided to rural areas in India.	951, 958	699, 701	J07, D08
3. Define primary health care. Write about staffing pattern and functioning of primary health center (PHC).	951, 964	699, 703	J14
4. Explain the concept of primary health care in India. List the functions of a primary health center.	958, 964	699, 704	D00, J02
5. Describe the set up and functions of a PHC.	964	703	J08
6. What is a "community health center"? Describe how health care is delivered to a population covered by a community development block.	967	709	D07(RS2)
Short Essays			
1. What are the determinants of primary health care?	—	700	J03
2. What is the role of non-governmental organizations (NGOs) in family planning?	—	—	D10
3. Discuss briefly about various levels (three-tier system) of health-care services and in brief its 'characteristics'.	950	699	J10(RS2), J12, D14
4. Define "primary health care". Write briefly about the "essential elements" and "guiding principles" of primary health care.	951	699	J12(RS2), D12(RS3), D14(RS3), J17(RS3), J18(RS3), J01, D02, D03, J04, D04, J11, D11, D12, D14, J17

Contd...

Contd...

	PARK	SYKNT	
5. Write the components of primary health care with examples.	951	700	D03
6. What is "appropriate technology"?	952	701	J07
7. Describe "ASHA"s role and responsibilities under National Rural Health Mission.	959	726	D12(RS3), J19(RS3)
8. Traditional birth attendant (Dai).	960	702	D06
9. Subcenter—health-care activites.	961	703	D01
10. Functions of a primary health center.	964	704	J03, J04, J05, D16
11. IPHS standards for staff pattern at primary health centre.	967	703	J19(RS3)
12. Describe a community health center—functions.	967	709	D11(RS2), D03, D10
13. Duties of medical officer in primary health center.	970	706	J09
14. Job description of multipurpose health worker (female).	971	707	D07(RS2), J09(RS2), J12(RS2), D13(RS3), D14(RS3), J05, D11
15. Job responsibilities of health workers (male).	973	707	J10, J14
16. Enumerate functions of health assistant (male).	975	708	D09
17. Central Government Health Scheme.	977	710	D18(RS3)
18. Name the three health schemes, which offers health insurance.	977	208	J04
19. Indigenous system of medicine.	978	710	J18(RS3)
20. Voluntary health agencies in India—define, enumerate and functions.	978	756	D11(RS2), D13(RS3), D00, J02
21. Briefly describe the role of NGOs in health care (non-governmental organization).	978	756	D10(RS2)
22. Write in short about Indian Red Cross (activities).	978	768	D00, J10
Short Answers			
1. Role of village health guides.	—	701	D02, D05

Contd...

COMMUNITY MEDICINE

Contd...

		PARK	SYKNT	
2.	How training of local dais is given?	—	702	J10(RS2)
3.	What is the duration of training of a local dai? What does she learn during her training?	—	702	J11(RS2)
4.	AYUSH in health-care services for the community.	—	710	J08(RS2)
5.	Write any voluntary organization working for de-addiction in India.	—	—	J11
6.	'Medical care' versus 'health care'	950	699	D15
7.	Describe the different levels of health-care delivery system in India.	950	699	D14(RS3), D13
8.	Primary health care—elements (components) and principles.	951	699	D13(RS3), J16(RS3), D16(RS3), D06, J06, J10
9.	Equitable distribution.	951	700	D15
10.	Define 'community participation' and give example.	951	700	J12
11.	Explain the term "appropriate technology" with examples.	951	701	J07, D08, J15
12.	What is HFA 2000 AD?	952	681	D00
13.	Accredited social health activist (ASHA)—job responsibilities.	959	726	J09(RS2), J17(RS3), D17(RS3)
14.	Describe the functions of subcenter.	961	703	J04
15.	List the ten functions of Primary health centers.	964	704	D02, J11
16.	Staff pattern of PHC.	967	703	J17
17.	Community health center.	967	709	D13(RS3), D17(RS3)
18.	What is the role of a health worker (male) as regards malaria eradication?	973	708	D10
19.	Central Government Health Scheme.	977	710	D11(RS2)
20.	Indigenous system of medicine.	978	710	D07(RS2), J09(RS2)
21.	Voluntary health organizations (NGOs)—enumerate (any six operating in India), role in health care.	978	756	D09(RS2), J18(RS3). J01, D06, J12

Contd...

Contd...

	PARK	SYKNT	
22. Indian Red Cross Society—activities.	978	768	D18(RS3), D11

CHAPTER 23
INTERNATIONAL HEALTH

Short Essays

1. Write briefly on World Food Day.	—	—	D11
2. World Health Organization (WHO) - functions/responsibilities.	982	760	J09(RS2), D11(RS2), J13(RS3), D14(RS3), D00, J02, D16
3. World Health Day (Theme 2012/2014).	982	760	J12
4. Role of World Health Organization in fields of biomedical research.	983	762	J02
5. Enumerate the international donor agencies and mention the activities of UNICEF in India.	985	763	J03, J11
6. Expand UNICEF. Describe activities of UNICEF (United Nations Children's Fund) in India—in child nutrition/Child health/improving child survival.	985	763	J08(RS2), J10(RS2), D12(RS3), J16(RS3), J19(RS3), J01, D01, D02, D04, J06, D12, J13, D13
7. Add a note on the United Nations Development Program.	986	764	D09
8. Food and agriculture organization (FAO).	986	764	D16(RS3)
9. Bilateral health agencies.	986	766	D18(RS3)
10. International Red Cross Society.	988	768	J08, J15

Short Answers

1. World Health Day (2003).	982	760	J04
2. List the activities of WHO.	983	761	D00, D02, D07
3. WHO role in disease control.	983	761	D05

Contd...

Contd...

		PARK	SYKNT	
4.	WHO—its role in health promotion.	983	761	J05
5.	World WHO regions and their headquarters.	984	760	J19(RS3), J02
6.	Enumerate functions of UNICEF.	985	763	D10(RS2)
7.	UNICEF—its role in child survival.	985	763	D03
8.	Expand GOBI (G O B I F F F).	985	764	D01, D04
9.	Write briefly on FAO (food and agriculture organization)—four aims.	986	764	J08
10.	List three purpose for which International Labor Organization (ILO) was established.	986	764	J01
11.	The Colombo Plan.	987	766	D18(RS3)
12.	Activities of SIDA in India.	987	766	J11
13.	Role of DANIDA in India.	987	766	J12
14.	Rockefeller foundation.	987	767	J09(RS2), J14
15.	CARE (functions in India).	987	768	J06, J09, D16
16.	International red cross society—activities/contribution.	988	768	J13(RS3), D15(RS3), D01, D04

MISCELLANEOUS

Short Essays

1.	Ring immunisation.	—	—	D13(RS3)
2.	Benefits of forming self-help groups of mothers in villages.	—	—	J08(RS2)
3.	What are the main health problems of urban slum dwellers and factors contributing to it?	—	—	J08(RS2)
4.	Vaccination for international travelers.	—	275	D07(RS2)

Short Answers

1.	Focus group discussion (FGD).	—	—	J15(RS3), D16(RS3)
2.	Screening for diseases in blood bank.	—	—	D07(RS2)
3.	List the demographic processes.	—	—	D07

Contd...

Contd...

		PARK	SYKNT	
4.	Slow viral diseases.	—	—	D07
5.	Attrition.	—	—	J11(RS2)
6.	Institute.	—	—	J11(RS2)
7.	Case definition for malaria.	—	—	D13(RS3)
8.	What are the guidelines for defining "at-risk" groups?	—	—	J15(RS3), D13
9.	Three measures of aging in a population.	—	—	D16
10.	Universal barrier precautions.	—	432	D07(RS2)
11.	Enumerate functions of a manager.	—	738	D10(RS2)

2

Ophthalmology

REFERENCES

1. AK Khurana, Aruj K Khurana, Bhawna Khurana **(KHRN)**: Comprehensive Ophthalmology, 7th Edition, Jaypee Brothers Medical Publishers (P) Ltd., New Delhi, ₹ 995/-
2. Samar K Basak **(BSAK)**: Essentials of Ophthalmology, 7th Edition, Jaypee Brothers Medical Publishers (P) Ltd., New Delhi, ₹ 895/-.

COURSE CONTENTS

THEORY

A. BASIC SCIENCES

I. Anatomy

- Development of the eye, coats of the eye, blood supply and nerve supply of the eye, pupillay pathways, visual pathways, extraocular muscles, oculomotor nerve.

II. Physiology

- Physiology of vision, tear film, aqueous humor formation.

III. Pharmacology

- Ophthalmic preparations and routes of administration
- Antibiotics, antivirals and antifungal drugs
- Cycloplegics, antiglaucoma drugs.

IV. Pathology

- Histopathology of retinoblastoma, malignant melanoma, squamous cell carcinoma, basal cell carcinoma.

V. Elementary Optics

- Reflection, refraction, optical system of normal eye, reduced eye, Sturm's conoid, estimation of refraction.

B. DISEASES OF EYE

I. Conjunctiva

Must Know

- Acute infective conjunctivitis
  - Bacterial conjunctivitis—purulent conjunctivitis, ophthalmia neonatorum, membranous conjunctivitis, chlamydial conjunctivitis—trachoma, viral conjunctivitis
- Allergic conjunctivitis
  - Simple, phlyctenular, vernal
- Conjunctival degenerations
  - Pterygium, pinguecula, concretions.

Desirable to Know

- Chronic conjunctivitis, inclusion conjunctivitis, pseudomembranous conjunctivitis
- Mucocutaneous diseases affecting conjunctiva
- Conjunctival tumors.

II. Cornea

Must Know

- Corneal ulcer
  - Etiology, clinical features, complications and treatment of bacterial, viral and fungal corneal ulcers
- Vitamin A deficiency and keratomalacia, exposure keratitis, neuroparalytic keratitis
- Interstitial keratitis
  - Etiology, clinical features and treatment
- Basics of eye donation and keratoplasty.

Desirable to Know

- Other forms of deep keratitis
- Degenerations of dystrophies of cornea, keratoconus
- Keratorefractive surgery.

III. Sclera

Must Know

- Episcleritis and scleritis
  - Clinical features, differential diagnosis, investigations and treatment.

Desirable to Know

- Scleromalacia perforans, blue sclera.

IV. Uveal Tract

Must Know

- Classification of uveitis
- Acute anterior uveitis
  - Etiology, clinical features, complications, differential diagnosis and management
- Purulent uveitis, endophthalmitis, panophthalmitis.

Desirable to Know

- Association of systemic diseases in uveitis
- Chronic uveitis, cyclitis, posterior uveitis
- Degenerative changes in the uveal tract
- Congenital anomalies
  - Coloboma of iris and choroids.

V. Lens

Must Know

- Classification of cataract
- Senile cataract
  - Etiology, clinical features and evaluation
  - Differential diagnosis from open angle glaucoma
  - Surgical management of cataract and complications of cataract surgery

- Aphakic corrections
- Intraocular lens implantation
- Congenital cataract—types
- Awareness of amblyopia, assessment and early reference
- Degeneration and opacities.

Desirable to Know

- Other forms of cataract
  - Complicated, traumatic, metabolic, toxic and after cataract
- Recent advances in cataract surgery—phacoemulsification.

VI. Vitreous

- Vitreous detachment, asteroid hyalosis, synchysis scintillans
- Vitreous hemorrhage
  - Causes and treatment.

VII. Glaucoma

Must Know

- Classification
- Angle closure glaucoma
  - Risk factors, mechanism, clinical features and management
  - Differential diagnosis of red eye
- Open angle glaucoma
  - Risk factors, cardinal signs, medical and surgical treatment
- Congenital glaucoma
  - Clinical features and management.

Desirable to Know

- Secondary glaucomas
  - Lens induced, inflammatory, neovascular, traumatic, intraocular tumors, steroid induced.

VIII. Retina

Must Know

- Fundus changes in:
  - Diabetes mellitus, hypertension, toxemia of pregnancy, renal diseases, hematological disease, AIDS, myopia
- Diabetic retinopathy
  - Risk factors, assessment and treatment, role of LASER photo-coagulation
- Retinal vascular diseases
  - CRAO (Central retinal artery occlusion), CRVO (Central retinal vein occlusion), Eale's disease
- Retinal detachment
  - Risk factors, clinical features, treatment.

Desirable to Know

- Retinal degeneration
  - Retinitis pigmentosa, familial lipid degenerations

- Retinal infections
  - Toxoplasma, toxocara, cytomegalovirus (CMV)
- Other
  - Phacomatosis.

IX. Optic Nerve

Must Know

- Papilledema
  - Etiology and fundus picture, differential diagnosis from papillitis
- Papillitis
  - Etiology and fundus picture
- Retrobulbar neuritis
- Optic atrophy
  - Primary, secondary, vascular, glaucomatous.

Desirable to Know

- Toxic amblyopia
- Optic nerve coloboma
- Intraocular tumors
- Retinoblastoma
  - Clinical features and treatment
  - Differential diagnosis of leukocoria
- Malignant melanoma
  - Clinical features and treatment.

X. Squint

- Classification
- Differentiation of paralytic and nonparalytic squint
- Types, etiology, assessment and principles of management of concomitant squint
- Awareness of amblyopia, assessment and early reference.

XI. Orbit

- Causes of proptosis
- Clinical features and treatment of orbital cellulitis and cavernous sinus thrombosis
- Common tumors of the orbit.

XII. Lacrimal System

- Causes of epiphora
- Etiology, clinical features, complications and management of congenital and acquired acute and chronic dacryocystitis
- Dry eye
  - Diagnosis and management.

XIII. Lids

- Inflammations
  - Blepharitis, hordeolum

- Anomalies in the position
  - Trichiasis, entropion, ectoprion, symblepharon, ankyloblepharon
- Lagophthalmos
- Ptosis
- Tumors of the lids.

XIV. Refractive Errors

Must Know

- Types, clinical presentation and optical corrections of myopia, hypermetropia, astigmatism, presbyopia, aphakia.

Desirable to Know

- Anisometropia, aniseikonia
- Anomalies of accommodation and convergence.

XV. Injuries

Must Know

- Perforating injuries
  - Mechanical effects, immediate and late complications including sympathetic ophthalmitis and endophthalmitis, immediate management and referral.
- Contusion injuries
  - Mechanical effects, delayed complications and referral
- Chemical burns
  - Immediate burns, immediate first aid, assessment and referral.

Desirable to Know

- Other forms of injuries, industrial, retained intraocular foreign body
- Medicolegal aspects of injuries.

XVI. Ophthalmic Surgery

- Cataract surgery
- Antiglaucoma operations
- Enucleation
- Evisceration
- Exenteration
- Dacryocystectomy
- Dacryocystorhinostomy.

XVII. Community Ophthalmology

- Definition and types of blindness
- Causes of blindness
- Objectives of NPCB and trachoma control project
- Organization of ophthalmic screening and cataract surgery camps.

XVIII. Miscellaneous

- Symptomatic disturbances of vision
  - Hemianopia, amblyopia, amaurosis, night blindness, color blindness, word blindness, malingering
- Ocular emergencies
  - Trauma, chemical burns, acute congestive glaucoma, endophthalmitis, sudden loss of vision
- Investigative ophthalmology
  - Ophthalmic ultrasound, computerized visual field testing, electroretinography, visual-evoked potential, CT scan
- Recent advances
  - Types and uses of LASER in ophthalmology.

CLINICAL

A. Skills

- Visual acuity test (use of pinhole)
- Color vision test
- Confrontation visual field test
- Cover test
- Ocular motility test
- Assessment of:
  - Corneal sensation Wick test
  - Corneal surface Placido's disk
  - Corneal ulcer Fluorescein staining
- Assessment of anterior chamber depth
- Papillary size and reaction
- Distant direct ophthalmoscopy for lens opacities
- Direct ophthalmoscopy.

B. Procedures (*These procedures are for observation only)

- Instillation of eye drops
- Irrigation of conjunctival sac
- Ophthalmic patch and bandage
- Epilation of eye lashes
- Eversion of upper eyelid
- Use of lid retractors to examine infant's eye*
- Lacrimal syringing test*
- Digital tonometry
- Use of Schiotz tonometer*
- Removal of extraocular foreign body*
- Subconjunctival injection*.

UNIVERSITY EXAMINATION PATTERN

Eligibility for Writing the University Examination

The candidate should have at least 35% aggregate in the two of the three internals conducted by the college and should also have minimum 75% attendance in Theory and Practical classes conducted.

Criteria for Passing the University Examination

The candidate should secure minimum 50% in the university theory examination (University theory + Viva voce) and the university practical examinations separately. Internal assessment marks would not be considered for passing criteria, however, they would be added to final marks to determine class of passing.

Distribution of Marks

	Internal Assessment		*University Examination*	
	Maximum marks	*Minimum marks to qualify*	*Maximum marks*	*Minimum marks to pass*
Theory examination	30 marks	11 marks	100 marks	60 marks
Viva voce	—	—	20 marks	
Practical examination	20 marks	07 marks	80 marks	40 marks

Distribution of Marks for University Examination

Theory Examination

It is of 150 marks in total, which consist of:

University Examination	100 marks
University Viva Voce	20 marks
Theory Internals	30 marks

Clinical Examination

It is of 100 marks in total, which consists of:

University Clinical	80 marks
Clinical Internals	20 marks

Theory Examination

There shall be one theory paper carrying 100 marks. The pattern of questions would be of three types.

2 Long Essay Questions	2 × 10 marks	20 marks
10 Short Essay Questions	10 × 5 marks	50 marks
10 Short Answer Questions	10 × 3 marks	30 marks
	Total	**100 marks**

Clinical Examination

Practical examination will carry 80 marks (2 cases of 40 marks each).

Viva Voce Examination

Viva voce carries 20 marks. And encompasses all aspects of syllabus and drugs and instruments.

Question Bank

	KHRN	BSAK	
Section I: Anatomy and Physiology of the Eye			
CHAPTER 1 **ANATOMY AND DEVELOPMENT OF THE EYE**			
Short Answer			
1. Mention the ocular coats of eye.	3	3	J08
CHAPTER 2 **PHYSIOLOGY OF EYE AND VISION**			
Short Answer			
1. Colour vision.	18	38	J17(RS3)
Section II: Optics and Refraction			
CHAPTER 3 **ELEMENTARY AND PHYSIOLOGICAL OPTICS**			
Short Answers			
1. Mention three uses of prisms in ophthalmology.	27	552	J06
2. Convex lenses—three uses.	28	551	J07
CHAPTER 4 **ERRORS OF REFRACTION AND ACCOMMODATION**			
Long Essays			
1. Describe the types and optical treatment of various refractive errors?	34	70	D13(RS2)
2. Define hypermetropia, discuss the etiology, types, clinical features and management of hypermetropia.	34	71	J12(RS2), D13
3. Define myopia. Discuss the etiology, types, symptoms/signs and management of myopia.	38	73	J14(RS2), J15(RS3), D16(RS3), D00, J03, J12
4. Discuss types/classification, etiology and management of astigmatism.	42	78	J19(RS3), D16

Contd...

OPHTHALMOLOGY

Contd...

	KHRN	BSAK	
Short Essays			
1. Classify refractive errors. Add a note on hypermetropia.	34	70	D18(RS3)
2. Hypermetropia—types, clinical presentation, complications and management (optical correction).	34	71	J08(RS2), J11(RS2), D17(RS3), J04, J16
3. Aphakia—define, causes, clinical features (signs), management/optical correction (unilateral aphakia), visual rehabilitation.	37	81	J10(RS2), D11(RS2), J16(RS3), J18(RS3), D02, D05, J10, D10, J17
4. Aphakic glasses—disadvantages.	37	83	J09
5. Pseudophakia.	38	—	D08(RS2), D06
6. Myopia—define, causes, clinical features, various modalities of correcting it.	38	73	D12(RS3), J13(RS3), J07, D07, J14, D14
7. Pathological (high) myopia—clinical features, fundus picture and management.	39	74	D08(RS2), D14(RS3), D01, J08, J15, D15
8. Draw a diagram of Sturm's conoid.	42	79	D08
9. Astigmatism—define, classify (diagram), modalities of correcting it.	42	78	J09(RS2), D10(RS2), D19(RS3), J02, J10, D12
10. Anisometropia.	44	85	J14
11. Presbyopia—define, causes, correction.	47	87	D09(RS2), D15(RS3), D02, D03, J08, J12, D12
12. What are the advantages and disadvantages of different types of lenses?	51	213	D09

Contd...

Contd...

		KHRN	BSAK	
13.	Describe the various uses of contact lens.	51	213	J14
14.	Describe the various type of surgeries performed to correct myopia.	52	76	J17
Short Answers				
1.	Accommodation.	45	86	D19(RS3)
2.	Draw the optical diagram of emmetropic, myopic and hypermetropic eye?	34, 38	70	D02
3.	Aphakia—causes, signs, spectacle correction.	37	81	J13(RS3), J14(RS2), D14(RS3)
4.	Describe the strum's conoid.	42	79	J13
5.	Anisometropia—define, three causes, two problems, significance.	44	85	D07(RS2), D10, J13
6.	Presbyopia.	47	87	J15(RS3)
7.	Bifocals.	50	88	D11(RS2), J16(RS3)
8.	Contact lenses—three advantages and disadvantages, indications, three complications.	50	212	D15(RS3), J01, J02, D04, D06, J08
9.	What is surgical treatment of myopia?	52	76	D03, D10
10.	Enumerate types of kerato refractive surgery.	52	76	J09
11.	Radial keratotomy.	52	76	J17(RS3)
12.	LASIK.	52	77	J08(RS2), D13(RS2), D15(RS3)

Section III: Diseases of Eye and Ocular Adnexa

CHAPTER 5
DISEASES OF CONJUNCTIVA

Long Essays

1.	Classify conjunctivitis. Discuss clinical features and management of trachoma.	61, 68	144, 155	J06, J15
2.	Discuss the differential diagnosis of acute conjunctivitis and how you manage a case of acute conjunctivitis.	63	145, 149	D08(RS2)

Contd...

Contd...

		KHRN	BSAK	
3.	Discuss etiology, clinical features, complication and management of ophthalmia neonatorum.	77	151	J14
4.	Discuss etiology, clinical features, complications and management of pterygium.	89	165	J10
Short Essays				
1.	Membranous conjunctivitis.	—	152	J10(RS2)
2.	Write briefly on phlycten.	—		D10(RS2), D08
3.	Describe the clinical features and management of purulent conjunctivitis.	63	150	J10
4.	Angular conjunctivitis (clinical features and management).	66	153	J13(RS3), D14(RS3), J06
5.	Trachoma—define, WHO classification, clinical (ocular) features, complications, treatment, SAFE, and control project.	67, 501	155	J09(RS2), D06, J07, J12, D13
6.	What is a pannus? Discuss causes of pannus. How do you treat pannus?	69	156	D09, D10
7.	Ophthalmia neonatorum.	77	151	D09(RS2), D13(RS2), J08
8.	Allergic conjunctivitis.	79	159	J19(RS3)
9.	Vernal keratoconjunctivitis (spring catarrh)—clinical features and management.	80	162	J08(RS2), J11(RS2), D11(RS2), J14(RS2), D14(RS3), D15(RS3), J16(RS3), D16(RS3), D17(RS3), D00, D01, D03, J11, D12, J13, D14

Contd...

Contd...

		KHRN	BSAK	
10.	Phlyctenular conjunctivitis/disease—clinical features and management.	84	160	J12(RS2), D19(RS3), J02, D06, D09
11.	Discuss pinguecula.	89	164	J14(RS2)
12.	Pterygium—define, treatment of recurrent pterygium (two agents used), surgical management (indications).	89	165	D09(RS2), J15(RS3), J04, D05, J12, D12, D15
13.	Differences between true and pseudopterygium.	90	166	D16
Short Answers				
1.	Tabulate differences between pseudo-membranous and membranous conjunctivitis.	—	147	D07
2.	Causes for pseudomembranous conjunctivitis.	—	148	J04
3.	Membranous conjunctivitis.	—	152	J17(RS3)
4.	Pannus.	69	156	J19(RS3)
5.	Phlycten.	—	160	D08(RS2)
6.	Herbert's pits.	69	156	D11(RS2), J16(RS3)
7.	Trachoma—three complication/six squeal/treatment.	70	155	J18(RS3), D01, D02, J05, J12, J14, J16
8.	Viral conjunctivitis—causes.	74	154	J09
9.	Ophthalmia neonatorum.	77	151	J12(RS2)
10.	Spring catarrh (Vernal-keratoconjunctivitis)—types/signs/treatment	81	162	D13(RS2), J16(RS3), J18(RS3), J04
11.	Pinguecula	89	164	J08(RS2)
12.	Pterygium (surgical management, three complications).	89	165	D15(RS3), J08, D15
13.	Pseudopterygium—define/causes.	90	166	D16(RS3), D06

Contd...

Contd...

		KHRN	BSAK	
14.	Define chemosis and ecchymosis. Mention two causes for each.	92	145	D02, J11
15.	What are the causes for subconjunctival hemorrhage and how is it managed?	92	171	J09(RS2), D12(RS3), J03, J05, J07, J09, D13, D16

CHAPTER 6
DISEASES OF CORNEA

Long Essays

1.	Define corneal ulcer. Mention the stages of corneal ulceration. Discuss the causes, clinical features, diagnosis, complications and management of a uncomplicated bacterial corneal ulcer (bacterial keratitis).	102	179	J13(RS3), J05, D07, D12
2.	Name three organisms which can penetrate intact corneal epithelium. Describe the etiopathogenesis, ocular manifestations (clinical features), investigation, complications and management of hypopyon corneal ulcer.	102, 105	179, 185	J08(RS2), D15(RS3), J18(RS3), J07, D10, D16
3.	Fungal keratitis/corneal ulcer (keratomycosis)—etiology, clinical features and management. Add a note on causes of non-healing corneal ulcer.	109, 108	187	J09(RS2), J19(RS3), J02, D03, J13
4.	Discuss various lesions of the cornea caused by herpes simplex. Add a note on treatment.	111	189	D08

Short Essays

1.	What are the factors responsible to protect the cornea against infection?	—	—	D11
2.	Describe ideal recipient for penetrating keratoplast.	—	—	J09
3.	Cornea—brief anatomy (mention layers).	98	3	D12(RS3), D03

Contd...

		KHRN	BSAK	
4.	Discuss factors for corneal transparency.	100	—	J17(RS3)
5.	Perforating corneal ulcer.	103	182	J12(RS2)
6.	Hypopyon corneal ulcer.	105	185	J14(RS2)
7.	Complications of corneal ulcer and sequelae of its perforation (complications of a perforated corneal ulcer).	106	181	J03, J11, J15, D15
8.	What is the role of atropine in the treatment of corneal ulcer? What alternative drug can be used in patients allergic to atropine? What drugs can be used if atropine fails to dilate the pupil?	108	185	D02
9.	Fungal corneal ulcer (fungal keratitis)—fungi responsible, clinical features, treatment (name two antifungal used in ophthalmology).	109, 468	187	D11(RS2), J15(RS3), J16(RS3), D08, D11, J16, J17
10.	Herpes simplex keratitis.	110	189	D09(RS2)
11.	Dendritic ulcer—clinical features and management.	111	190	J18(RS3), D18(RS3), D01, J11, D14
12.	Herpes zoster ophthalmicus—ocular manifestations, complications and management.	113	192	J01, D04
13.	Acanthamoeba keratitis.	116	189	D07(RS2), J11(RS2), J13(RS3), D17(RS3)
14.	Neuroparalytic keratitis—etiology, clinical features and treatment.	118	194	D10
15.	Exposure keratitis (causes and management).	119	194	D08(RS2), D13
16.	Peripheral ulcerative keratitis (PUK)—management.	120	195	D16(RS3)
17.	Mooren's ulcer—clinical features and treatment.	120	196	D00

Contd...

Contd...

		KHRN	BSAK	
18.	What are causes of deep keratitis? Interstitial keratitis—stages, clinical features, management.	124	199	D02, D06, J08, D09
19.	Arcus senilis—diagnostic criteria.	126	201	J09
20.	Keratoconus.	135	206	D16
21.	Corneal edema.	137	177	D11(RS2), J16(RS3)
22.	Corneal opacity—treatment.	138	—	D19(RS3)
23.	Keratoplasty—types, indication (penetrating keratoplasty)and contraindications. Add a note on eyebank.	141, 509	488, 493	J04, D05, D08, J13
Short Answers				
1.	Layers of cornea—list/draw a labeled diagram.	99	4	J10(RS2), J14(RS2), J06
2.	What is the nerve supply of cornea? Give two causes for diminished corneal sensation.	99	5	D05
3.	What are the stages of corneal ulcer?	103	179	J04
4.	What is hypopyon? Give three causes for hypopyon corneal ulcer.	105	185	D05
5.	Sequel of corneal ulcer perforation.	106	182	J12
6.	Corneal scars.	106	180	J18(RS3)
7.	Atropine sulfate 1% in corneal ulcer.	108	185	D14
8.	Mention features of fungal hypopyon,	110	188	J09
9.	Name two investigations for fungal corneal ulcer. Mention two topical and two systemic antifungal agents.	110	188	J14
10.	Herpes simplex—corneal signs.	111	190	D10(RS2)
11.	Herpes zoster ophthalmicus—ocular manifestations.	113	192	D12
12.	Exposure ketarititis and treatment.	119	194	D13(RS2), D14
13.	Mooren's ulcer.	120	196	J17(RS3)
14.	Enumerate features of corneal dystrophies.	128	203	D07

Contd...

Contd...

		KHRN	BSAK	
15.	Keratoconus—signs.	135	206	J15(RS3), D16(RS3), J10
16.	Corneal opacity—three grades.	138	177	D14(RS3)
17.	What is anterior staphyloma?	138	182	D06
18.	Keratoplasty (indications).	141	488	J11(RS2), J12(RS2), D16(RS3), D17(RS3), D18(RS3), D03, J12, J15
19.	Penetrating keratoplasty (indications).	141	488	D08(RS2), D11(RS2), J16(RS3)
20.	Paracentesis—three indications.	—	487	J01, D04

CHAPTER 7
DISEASES OF SCLERA

Short Essays

		KHRN	BSAK	
1.	Episcleritis—define, causes, signs and symptoms and its management. How do you differentiate episcleritis and scleritis?	146	215	D08(RS2), J11(RS2), J13(RS3), J16(RS3), D17(RS3), J06, D10
2.	Scleritis (classify, clinical features, systemic association, management).	147	216	J08(RS2), D16(RS3), D06, D07, J13
3.	Scleromalacia perforans.	148	217	D11
4.	What is sclera and staphyloma? Staphyloma—define, classify, causes, treatment.	149	—	D00, D10, D16

Short Answers

		KHRN	BSAK	
1.	Episcleritis.	146	215	J14(RS2)
2.	Deep scleritis.	147	216	D15(RS3)
3.	Scleromalacia perforans.	148	217	D09, D14
4.	Mention complication of scleritis.	149	—	J12

Contd...

Contd...

		KHRN	BSAK	
5.	Staphyloma.	149	—	J19(RS3)
6.	Classify staphylomas.	149	—	J16, J17
7.	Mention causes of posterior staphyloma.	150	—	D07

CHAPTER 8
DISEASES OF UVEAL TRACT

Long Essays

1.	Discuss clinical features and complications of chronic iridocyclitis.	158	226	D11(RS2), J16(RS3)
2.	Discuss the etiology, clinical features and management of granulomatous iridocyclitis.	158, 164	235	J09(RS2)
3.	Discuss the differential diagnosis of acute red eye. Classify uveitis and discuss etiopathogenesis, classification, clinical features, sequel and complications and management of acute iridocyclitis.	163, 155, 158	224	D09(RS2), D10(RS2), J17(RS3), D19(RS3), J01, D04, J10, D11, D15
4.	Enumerate causes of red eye. Discuss the symptoms, signs and management of anterior uvetitis.	163, 158	226	D18(RS3)
5.	Classify endophthalmitis and discuss the clinical features and management of acute postoperative endophthalmitis.	176	243	D14

Short Essays

1.	Pars planitis—complication.	—	231	J09
2.	Classify uveitis and add note on principles of management of acute iridocyclitis.	155, 164	224, 231	J06
3.	Acute iritis/iridocyclitis.	158	226	D16(RS3), J19(RS3)
4.	Granulomatus uveitis (iridocyclitis).	158	235	J08(RS2), J12(RS2), J16
5.	Acute anterior uveitis (iridocyclitis)—clinical signs, investigations and its management (of recurrent uveitis).	159	226	J15(RS3), D01, J03, D03, D13

Contd...

Contd...

		KHRN	BSAK	
6.	What are keratic precipitates? What are the different types of keratic precipitates.	159	226	J13(RS3)
7.	What do the terms occlusive pupillae and seclusio pupillae denote?	161	229	D02
8.	Occlusio pupillae.	162	229	D14(RS3)
9.	What is rubeosis iridis? Mention its causes and complications.	162	228	D01
10.	Discuss the effect of anterior uveitis on intraocular pressure.	162	229	D00
11.	Discuss the mechanism of glaucoma in a patient with uveitis.	162	230	D07(RS2)
12.	Phthisis bulbi.	163	230	J15(RS3)
13.	Describe features of granulomatous and non-granulomatous uveitis.	164	226	J11
14.	What are the differences between granulomatous and non-granulomatous uveitis?	164	226	J01, D04, J12, J15, J17
15.	What are the pharmacological effects of atropine in the eye? Mention its uses.	164	231	J01, J02, D04
16.	(Acute bacterial postoperative) endophthalmitis—clinical features, management.	176	243	J10(RS2), D05, D12, J13
17.	Panophthalmitis.	178	244	D08(RS2), J04, D10
18.	Evisceration—indications and technique.	178	499	D07(RS2), D06, J13, J14
19.	Malignant melanoma of choroid (clinical features).	180	374	J12(RS2), D07
Short Answers				
1.	Ciliary zone is called the "danger zone of eye". Explain.	—	239	J02
2.	Describe the differences between endophthalmitis and panophthalmitis.	—	—	J14
3.	Differences between enucleation and evisceration.	—	—	D13(RS2)
4.	Enumerate parts of uveal tract.	151	8	J09

Contd...

Contd...

		KHRN	BSAK	
5.	Coloboma of iris.	154	221	J08(RS2)
6.	Mention three syndromes associated with uveitis?	156	225	J02
7.	What are the features of granulomatous uvetis?	158	226	J14
8.	Keratic precipitates—three types.	159	226	J07
9.	Aqueous flare and its detection.	160	226	J13(RS3)
10.	Occlusive and seclusive papillae.	161	229	J12(RS2), J18(RS3)
11.	Rubeosis iridis—causes and complications.	162	228	D02
12.	Mention the causes of glaucoma in iridocyclitis.	162	230	D11
13.	Phthysis bulbi.	163	230	J18(RS3)
14.	Management of acute anterior uveitis.	164	231	J11(RS2), D17(RS3)
15.	Mention three differences between granulomatous and non-granulomatous uveitis .	164	226	J08
16.	VKH syndrome.	175	238	J10(RS2)
17.	Evisceration—define, two/three indications.	178	499	D08(RS2), D14(RS3), D08, D14, D16

CHAPTER 9
DISEASES OF LENS

Long Essays

1.	Define cataract. Classify cataract. Describe the types, stages of senile cataract. Discuss clinical features of senile cataract and its management with recent developments. Add a note on phacoemulsification.	187, 193, 202, 211	256, 262, 474	J13(RS3), J17(RS3), J08, D10, J12, J14
2.	Congenital/developmental cataract—classification, etiology, morphological type, clinical features, management and complications.	188	257	D09(RS2), J14(RS2), J02, J04, J17
3.	Cortical cataract—etiology, symptoms and stages.	193	263	D15(RS3)

Contd...

OPHTHALMOLOGY

Contd...

		KHRN	BSAK	
4.	Senile immature cataract—etiology, clinical features and management.	194	263	J11(RS2), D17(RS3)
5.	Discuss the clinical features and management of senile mature cataract. Add a note on early complications of cataract surgery.	194, 202, 219	264, 481	D13
6.	Discuss the complications of senile cataract. How will you manage them?	199	266	D00
7.	Discuss the preoperative assessment done for cataract surgery.	202	269	J03
8.	Classify types of cataract surgeries. Describe the surgical procedure of manual small incision cataract surgery.	204, 208	273, 472	D14(RS3)
9.	Describe and compare the various types of cataract surgeries?	204	470	D13(RS2)
Short Essays				
1.	Congenital cataract (management).	188	257	D16(RS3), J13
2.	Discuss the causes of cataract in patients under 30 years of age.	188	258	J05
3.	Zonular cataract.	189	260	D07(RS2), D08(RS2), J01, D04
4.	Discuss the complications due to hypermature cataract.	199	266	J09(RS2)
5.	Complicated cataract—define, causes and clinical features.	200	275	J08(RS2), J12(RS2), D12(RS3), J18(RS3), J19(RS3), J07, J11, J15, D16
6.	What are the investigations done before cataract surgery?	202	269	D03
7.	Discuss various macular function tests?	203	272	D05
8.	Describe the advantages of conventional extracapsular cataract extractions (ECCE) over intracapsular cataract extraction (ICCE).	204	478	J17

Contd...

Contd...

		KHRN	BSAK	
9.	Describe the differences between conventional extracapsular cataract extraction (ECCE) from phacoemulsification.	205	274	J13
10.	Discuss the advantages and disadvantages of phacoemulsification.	205	275	D14
11.	Intraocular lens (IOL)—define, types, advantages.	213	477	J12(RS2), D02
12.	Intraocular lens power calculation.	216	270	D16(RS3)
13.	Describe the complications of extracapsular cataract extraction.	217	482	J16
14.	Postoperative complications of cataract surgery.	219	481	D16(RS3)
15.	Hyphema—define, causes, complications and its management.	219	445	D12(RS3), J17(RS3), D19(RS3), J02, D08, J11, J17
16.	After cataract.	221	277	D13(RS2)
17.	Ocular manifestation of Marfan's syndrome.	222	254	J06
Short Answers				
1.	What is 'TORCH' test?	—	261	J09
2.	Crystalline lens—parts, draw and label.	184	11	D15(RS3), J18(RS3), J15
3.	Nuclear cataract.	194	266	J12(RS2)
4.	Mention the clinical stages of senile cortical cataract.	194	267	J15
5.	Symptoms of senile immature cataract.	194	268	D14(RS3)
6.	Morgagnian cataract.	195	265	D08(RS2)
7.	Mention three signs of hypermature cataract.	195	268	D01, J11
8.	Explain what is second vision (Second sight).	196	267	D09(RS2), J14
9.	Metabolic cataract.	199	276	J10(RS2)

Contd...

Contd...

		KHRN	BSAK	
10.	Mention the conditions in which following cataract occur.			
	a. Sunflower cataract.	200	457	D02
	b. Rosette cataract.	448	448	
	c. Occupational cataract.	201	277	
	d. Snow flake cataract.	199	276	
	e. After cataract.	221	277	
	f. Complicated cataract.	200	275	
11.	Complicated cataract—causes, clinical features.	200	275	D16(RS3), D07, J10, D13, D14
12.	Name different types of anesthesia used for cataract surgery.	204	467	D10
13.	Advantages of phacoemulsifications?	205	275	J09(RS2), D16(RS3), D18(RS3), J01, D04
14.	Mention three advantages of small incision cataract surgery.	205	274	J07
15.	Describe the differences between phacoemulsification and conventional extracapsular cataract extraction?	205	274	D12
16.	Types of extracapsular cataract extraction.	206	273	J19(RS3)
17.	Small incision cataract surgery.	208	274	J14(RS2)
18.	What is phacoemulsificaition?	211	275	D19(RS3), J05
19.	Name different types of intraocular lenses.	213	478	D08
20.	What are the differences between AC-IOL and PC-IOL?	213	479	J10
21.	Name various materials used in manufacturing of intraocular lens.	214	480	D07(RS2)
22.	Types of PC-IOL.	214	479	D15
23.	IOL power calculation.	216	270	D09(RS2)
24.	What is SRK formula?	216	271	J13
25.	Enumerate preoperative complications of cataract surgery.	217	—	D07

Contd...

Contd...

		KHRN	BSAK	
26.	What are the complications following vitreous loss during cataract surgery?	218	481	J02
27.	Mention three complications of extracapsular cataract extraction.	218	482	J14
28.	Hypheama—define, causes, complications.	219	445	J09(RS2), J18(RS3), J09
29.	Mention late (delayed) complications of cataract surgery.	220	482	D05
30.	After cataract (posterior capsule opacity)—define, types, treatment.	221	277	D07(RS2), J08(RS2), J15(RS3), D06, D08
31.	Mention intraocular lens related complications.	221	479	J15
32.	Subluxation of the lens—four causes/ three syndromes associated.	223	279	J06, D11

CHAPTER 10
GLAUCOMA

Long Essays

1.	Classify glaucomas and discuss about clinical features and management of congenital glaucoma.	231, 233	287	J08, J15
2.	Enumerate the causes for gradual loss of vision. Primary open angle glaucoma/chronic simple glaucoma—etiology, risk factors, pathogenesis, clinical features, field defects, diagnosis and management (medical/ drugs used).	514, 236	264, 298	J10(RS2), J18(RS3), D19(RS3), J07, J11, J17
3.	Acute primary angle closure glaucoma—etiology, predisposing/ risk factors, clinical features and treatment (of acute attack).	246, 251	289	D10(RS2), J12(RS2), J15(RS3), J13, D14

Short Essays

1.	Mechanism of primary and secondary angle closure glaucoma.	—	289, 299, 311	D11(RS2), J16(RS3)
2.	Draw and label a diagram of aqueous outflow from the eye.	227	282	D00, J12

Contd...

Contd...

		KHRN	BSAK	
3.	Describe circulation of aqueous humor.	229	30	J09
4.	Factors responsible for maintenance of intra-ocular pressure.	229	282	J19(RS3)
5.	Buphthalmos (congenital/infantile glaucoma)—clinical feature and management.	232	287	D08(RS2), D10(RS2), J11(RS2), D13(RS2), D17(RS3), J04, J06, J10, D13
6.	Primary open angle glaucoma/ chronic simple glaucoma—optic disc changes, visual field defects, medical management.	236	298	D11(RS2), J14(RS2), J01, J02, D03, D04, D09, D11, D15, J16
7.	Topical drugs in glaucoma.	243	308	J10(RS2)
8.	Angle closure (narrow angle) glaucoma—causes, clinical stages, clinical features and treatment (acute congestive attack).	246	289, 296	D18(RS3), J04, J05, D05, J14
9.	Iris bombe.	247	229	D15(RS3)
10.	Acute congestive glaucoma (clinical features, management and differential diagnosis).	251	290	J08(RS2), D15(RS3), D01, J03
11.	Chronic congestive glaucoma.	253	292	D09(RS2)
12.	What is absolute glaucoma?	254	292	J04, J12
13.	How do you recognize and treat secondary glaucoma due to hypermature cataract?	254	312	D03
14.	Lens induced glaucoma (LIG)—clinical features and treatment.	254	311	D18(RS3), J09
15.	Phacolytic glaucoma.	255	312	J15(RS3), D08
16.	Neovascular glaucoma—etiologyandclinical features.	257	314	J09(RS2)
17.	Pseudoexfoliation syndrome/ glaucoma.	257	311	J09(RS2), J18(RS3), D10

Contd...

Contd...

		KHRN	BSAK	
18.	Iridectomy—indications and complications.	260	486	J17(RS3), J10
19.	Trabeculectomy—indications and mention any two additional agents used to prevent its failure.	261	483	J14
Short Answers				
1.	Optical iridectomy.	—	487	J10(RS2)
2.	How is aqueous humor formed?	228	30	D09(RS2), D03
3.	Congenital glaucoma (buphthalmos)—management.	234	287	D09, D14
4.	Optic disc changes in glaucoma.	237	300	D13(RS2)
5.	Typical field defects/visual field changes of primary open angle glaucoma.	240	303	D12(RS3), J10
6.	Mention provocative tests for open angle glaucoma.	242	295	D05
7.	Iris bombe (define, two causes).	247	229	J15(RS3), D08
8.	Mention stages of narrow angle glaucoma (primary angle closure glaucoma).	249	290	J09, J12
9.	Mention three topical drugs and their mechanism of action in treatment of primary angle closure glaucoma.	252	308	D12
10.	Glaukomflecken.	253	291	D11(RS2)
11.	Give three causes for secondary glaucoma.	254	311	D09
12.	What are lens-induced glaucomas?	254	311	J16
13.	Mention three causes for neovascular glaucoma.	257	314	J03, J11, J15
14.	Discuss the mechanism of steroid-induced glaucoma.	258	316	J09(RS2)
15.	Indications of peripheral iridectomy.	260	486	D03
16.	Mention uses of mitomycin C in eye.	261	311	D16(RS3)
17.	Mention two cyclodestructive procedures. What are the associated complications?	263	—	D12

Contd...

Contd...

	KHRN	BSAK	
CHAPTER 11 **DISEASES OF VITREOUS**			
Short Essays			
1. Asteroid hyalosis.	267	322	D10
2. Vitreous hemorrhage—causes, management.	268	323	J19(RS3), J02, D12
Short Answers			
1. Types of vitreous opacities.	267	321	D18(RS3)
2. Asteroid hyalosis.	267	322	D08(RS2), J11(RS2), D17(RS3)
3. Synchysis scintillans.	267	322	J08(RS2)
4. Vitreous hemorrhage—mention three causes and three complications.	268	323	D01, D02, J04, D13, J16
CHAPTER 12 **DISEASES OF RETINA**			
Long Essays			
1. (Proliferative) diabetic retinopathy—define, ETDR's classification, clinical features and management.	285	352	D16(RS3), D18(RS3), D12
2. Rhegmatogenous retinal detachment—clinical features, risk factors and management.	309	345	J11(RS2), D17(RS3)
3. What is leukocoria? Enumerate the causes for the same (differential diagnosis of amaurotic cats eye reflex in a child). Describe retinoblastoma in detail (management).	317, 314	382, 378	J08(RS2), J16
Short Essays			
1. Eale's disease.	276	323	J17(RS3)
2. Central retinal artery occlusion (fundus picture).	277	333	D07(RS2), J08(RS2), J06, D08, J14, D14
3. (Ischemic) central retinal vein occlusion—fundus picture/two complications.	279	335	J13(RS3), J01, J02, D04, J11, D12, J13, J16

Contd...

OPHTHALMOLOGY

Contd...

		KHRN	BSAK	
4.	Hypertensive retinopathy—classify/Stages, fundus picture (ophthalmoscopic appearance) in each stage (Grade III).	281	350	D08(RS2), J09(RS2), D10(RS2), J14(RS2), D14(RS3), J17(RS3), J19(RS3), D02, J04, J05, D05, D07, J10
5.	(Proliferative) diabetic retinopathy (clinical features/fundus picture/ complications/treatment).	285	352	D09(RS2), D12(RS3), D13(RS2), J15(RS3), D00, D06, J07, D09, D13, D14, J15, D15, D16
6.	Retinitis pigmentosa—etiology, different types, clinical features, fundus picture.	296	342	D10(RS2), J15(RS3), D19(RS3), D09, J13, J17
7.	(Rhegmatogenous) retinal detachment—define, classify, clinical features and management.	309	345	J10(RS2), D11(RS2), D12(RS3), J15(RS3), J16(RS3), J16
8.	Retinoblastoma—clinical stages, histopathology, clinical presentation, management.	314	378	D11(RS2), J16(RS3), J17(RS3), D19(RS3), D05, D11
9.	Differential diagnosis of amaurotic cat's eye reflex.	317	382	D15(RS3)
10.	Enucleation—indications, contra-indications, procedure (steps) for enucleations.	320	499	J09(RS2), D14(RS3), J03, J10, J11, D13

Short Answers

1.	What are the layers of the retina?	272	12	D08(RS2), D19(RS3), D06, D15

Contd...

Contd...

		KHRN	BSAK	
2.	Fundus picture of central retinal artery occlusion.	277	333	D03
3.	Mention four signs in hypertensive retinopathy.	282	351	D12(RS3)
4.	Discuss fundus picture in diabetic retinopathy.	287	354	J11(RS2), D17(RS3)
5.	Retinitis pigmentosa (three diagnostic signs/three systemic associations).	296	342	J12(RS2), D16(RS3), J03, J04, J11, J15
6.	Photoretinitis.	301	—	D09(RS2)
7.	Classify retinal detachment. Mention three surgical modalities in the treatment of retinal detachment.	309	345	J13(RS3), D05, D09, D12
8.	Three causes for retinal detachment.	309	345	J05
9.	Mention two causes for exdudative retinal detachment.	312	345	D12(RS3)
10.	Retinoblastoma—stages, histopathology, clinical features, treatment.	314	379	D07(RS2), D08(RS2), J19(RS3), J01, D04, D09, J10, D13, J15
11.	Sturge-Weber syndrome—define/ features.	320	378	J04, D11
12.	Enucleation (indications).	320	499	J08(RS2), J11(RS2), D17(RS3), J05, J06

CHAPTER 13 NEURO-OPHTHALMOLOGY

Long Essays

1.	Describe the pathway of the pupillary light reflex. Discuss normal and abnormal reactions of the pupil.	327	44	D09
2.	What are the causes for sudden loss of vision in adults? What is the etiology, stages, fundus picture and differential diagnosis of papilledema?	514, 336	366	D07(RS2), D03

Contd...

Contd...

	KHRN	BSAK	
Short Essays			
1. Write visual pathway (draw diagram).	322	43	D18(RS3), D16
2. Hemianopia.	326	43	D13(RS2)
3. Draw and label a diagram of pupillary pathways.	327	45	D01
4. Draw a neat labeled diagram of light reflex pathway.	327	45	D13
5. Marcus gunn pupil (afferent pupillary defect).	328	45	D11(RS2), J16(RS3), J17(RS3)
6. Optic neuritis—signs, symptoms, optic disc changes and management.	329	362	J11(RS2), D15(RS3), D17(RS3), J09
7. Papillitis.	330	362	D01, J04
8. Retrobulbar neuritis—clinical features and management.	330	362	J10(RS2), D14
9. Tobacco amblyopia—clinical features.	332	364	D07
10. Papilledema (clinical features/fundus picture).	336	366	D08(RS2), J12(RS2), J03, J12, J15
11. What are the fundus changes in intracranial space occupying lesions?	337	368	D09
12. Optic atrophy (classify with examples and one cause for each type).	338	370	D09(RS2), D16(RS3), D02, D07
13. How will you differentiate papillitis from papilledema?	339	369	J07, D08, D13, J16
14. Describe the fundus picture in primary optic atrophy. Name two causes of primary optic atrophy.	340	370	D11
15. Night blindness.	341	511	D09(RS2)
16. Color blindness.	342	40	J14(RS2), J19(RS3)
Short Answers			
1. Tubular vision—two causes.	—	—	D14(RS3), J17(RS3), J03, J04, J11

Contd...

Contd...

		KHRN	BSAK	
2.	Visual pathway (draw and label).	322	43	J08(RS2), J17
3.	What is Marcus Gunn pupil? Mention three conditions.	328	45	D10(RS2), D05, D10
4.	Argyll Robertson pupil.	329	46	J10(RS2), D14(RS3)
5.	Adie's pupil.	329	46	J11(RS2), D17(RS3)
6.	Six causes of chronic retrobulbar neuritis.	330	362	D10(RS2)
7.	What are the diagnostic criteria for acute retrobulbar neuritis?	330	363	J01, J02, D04
8.	Mention two signs of optic neuritis.	330	363	D12(RS3)
9.	Toxic amblyopia.	332	364	J08(RS2)
10.	Mention the causes of toxic optic neuropathy.	332	364	J13
11.	Define papilledema.	336	366	J09
12.	Mention three causes of optic disc edema.	336	367	J14
13.	Types of optic atrophy.	338	370	J14, D16
14.	Differences between primary and secondary optic atrophy.	338	370	J04
15.	Three causes for optic atrophy.	340	370	D03
16.	Primary optic atrophy—causes/optic disc changes.	340	370	J14(RS2), J15(RS3)
17.	Secondary optic atrophy—causes and fundus appearance.	340	370	D10(RS2), J12
18.	Consecutive optic atropy—define, two causes.	340	370	J10(RS2), D00
19.	Nyctalopia (night blindness)—define, four causes.	341	511	D07(RS2), D19(RS3), D05, D07, J08, D12, D13
20.	Color blindness—classify/testing.	342	40	D07(RS2), J15(RS3), D08
21.	Amaurosis fugax.	343	334	D15

Contd...

Contd...

		KHRN	BSAK	
22.	Two tests for malingering.	344	—	D12(RS3)
23.	Name three demyelinating diseases.	347	—	J19(RS3)

CHAPTER 14
DISORDERS OF OCULAR MOTILITY

Long Essay

		KHRN	BSAK	
1.	Classify squint. Discuss clinical features, investigation and management of paralytic squint.	358, 367	425, 433	J06, D07

Short Essays

		KHRN	BSAK	
1.	Mention the names of extraocular muscles and its actions.	349	16, 418	J07, J15
2.	Amblyopia—definition, causes and treatment.	355	424	D10(RS2), D14(RS3)
3.	What is anisometropic amblyopia? How do you treat it?	356	424	D03
4.	Concomitant squint—clinical features and assessment/investigations.	361	427	D15(RS3), D07
5.	Paralytic squint.	367	433	J08(RS2)
6.	Differentiation between paralytic (concomitant) and nonparalytic (incomitant) squint?	371	434	J09(RS2), D18(RS3), J03, D05, D10, J12
7.	What are the principles of squint surgery? What are the causes of convergent squint?	372	431	J05

Short Answers

		KHRN	BSAK	
1.	What are the elevators of upper lid? Mention their nerve supply.	—	18	D01
2.	Extraocular muscles—names, nerve supply, actions.	349	16	D09(RS2), J12(RS2), J13(RS3), D14(RS3), D18(RS3), J02, J03, D05
3.	Superior oblique muscle—origin, insertion, nerve supply, three actions.	349	16	D07(RS2), D03, J05, D09, J11

Contd...

Contd...

		KHRN	BSAK	
4.	Superior rectus muscle—nerve supply, actions.	349	16	D10
5.	What are the depressors of eye? Mention their nerve supply.	349	16	J12
6.	Amblyopia—classify, etiology, significance.	355	424	J09(RS2), D11(RS2), J16(RS3)
7.	Classify diplopia. Give one example for each of them.	357	422	D08
8.	What is pseudosquint? Give two examples.	358	425	J01, D04
9.	Classification of squint.	358	426	D19(RS3)
10.	Mention two tests to measure the amount of squint.	359	430	D11
11.	Mention the methods and management of concomitant squint?	364	431	D01
12.	Hirschberg test.	365	430	J13(RS3)
13.	Paralytic squint—causes, features (signs).	367	433	J14(RS2), J06, J13
14.	Differences between concomitant (paralytic) and incomitant (non-paralytic) squints.	371	434	D14
15.	Name the weakening procedures to correct squint.	372	431	J09(RS2)
16.	What is nystagmus? Name two causes of nystagmus.	373	440	D10

CHAPTER 15
DISEASES OF EYELIDS

Short Essays

1.	Anatomy of eye lid.	377	17	J18(RS3)
2.	Blepharitis (causes, clinical manifestations and its treatment).	380	135	J08(RS2), D13(RS2), J17(RS3), J07, J08
3.	Ulcerative blepharits—clinical features, complications and treatment.	380	136	D01, J11
4.	Squamous blepharitis.	381	135	D14(RS3)

Contd...

Contd...

		KHRN	BSAK	
5.	Hordeolum externum (stye)—define, causes, clinical features and management.	383	138	J14(RS2), D05, D07
6.	Chalazion—etiology, clinical features, complications and management.	383	139	J15(RS3), J02, J03, J06, J11
7.	Trichiasis—define, causes, treatment.	385	126	D00
8.	Entropion—classify, causes, management.	387	121	D19(RS3), J05, D09, D10
9.	Senile ectropion.	390	124	D08
10.	Symblepharon—define, causes and its management.	392	127	D12(RS3), J17(RS3)
11.	Lagophthalmos (causes, complications and treatment).	393	127	J12(RS2), J01, D04, D06, J16
12.	Tarsorrhaphy—indications, steps.	394	495	D08, D12
13.	Ptosis—define, classify, causes, correction.	395	130	D12(RS3), D16(RS3), D02, D06, J09, J15, D15

Short Answers

1.	Draw and label a diagram of the cross section of the upper eyelid.	378	19	J01, D02, J03, D04, J08
2.	Ulcerative blepharitis (complications).	380	136	J16
3.	Hordeolum externum (clinical features and management).	383	138	J09(RS2), D12(RS3), D14(RS3), D13
4.	Chalazion [define, management (operation), complications].	383	139	D11(RS2), J12(RS2), J16(RS3), J18(RS3), D18(RS3), D19(RS3), D06, J13, D16
5.	Hordeolum internum.	385	140	D07(RS2), J10(RS2)

Contd...

Contd...

		KHRN	BSAK	
6.	Trichiasis (two causes).	385	126	D12(RS3), J10
7.	Cicatricial entropion—three causes.	387	123	D14
8.	Ectropion—classification.	389	124	J17
9.	Symblepharon (define, two causes).	392	127	D07(RS2), J08(RS2), J19(RS3), D09, J12, J15
10.	Lagophthalmus (etiology and management).	393	127	J11(RS2), J17(RS3), D17(RS3)
11.	Tarsorrhaphy—define, four indications.	394	495	D01
12.	Ptosis (define and classify/three causes/treatment).	395	130	J13(RS3), D15(RS3), J19(RS3), D03, J11, D12, D16
13.	What is Marcus Gunn jaw winking phenomenon?	395	130	J05
14.	Horner's syndrome—signs (ocular components).	395	47	D10(RS2), D12(RS3), J17(RS3), J01, D04, D15

CHAPTER 16
DISEASES OF LACRIMAL APPARATUS

Long Essays

1.	Discuss the causes of watering in the eye. How will you investigate a case of epiphora?	408	410	D01
2.	Chronic dacryocystitis—define, etiology, clinical features, complications and (surgical) management. Add a note on anatomy of the nasolacrimal apparatus.	411, 402	414, 20	D08(RS2), D12(RS3), D14(RS3), D05, D06, J16
3.	Acute dacryocystitis—define, etiology, clinical manifestations, complications and treatment.	412	414	J09, J11

Contd...

Contd...

	KHRN	BSAK	
4. Dacryocystectomy—define, indications, steps of surgery.	415	497	D02
Short Essays			
1. Normal anatomy of lacrimal passages.	404	20	D13(RS2)
2. Tear film—layers and their functions.	404	28	D07(RS2)
3. Dry eye—causes, diagnosis and management.	406	403	J11(RS2), D17(RS3), D15(RS3), J05, D07
4. Schirmer's test—indication, procedure and interpretation.	407	407	D10(RS2)
5. Epiphora.	408	410	J14(RS2)
6. Congenital dacryocystitis (naso-lacrimal duct obstruction)—aetiology, clinical features, complications and treatment.	410	415	J09(RS2), D10(RS2), D00, J03, D11, J12, J14, D14
7. Chronic dacryocystitis (clinical features and management).	411	414	J02, J08
8. Acute dacryocystitis—clinical features, treatment and complications.	412	414	J10(RS2), J18(RS3), J01, D03, J04, D04, J05
9. Discuss principle of dacryocysto–rhionostomy.	413	498	J04
Short Answers			
1. Dacryocystectomy (DCT)—indications	—	417	D16
2. Tear film—layers (constituents)and functions	404	28	D08(RS2), D11(RS2), J13(RS3), D13(RS2), J16(RS3), D01, J07, D09, J12
3. Epiphora—define, 3 causes.	408	410	D09(RS2), D08

Contd...

Contd...

		KHRN	BSAK	
4.	Congenital dacryocystitis.	410	415	D19(RS3)
5.	Chronic dacryocystitis.	411	414	D15(RS3)
6.	Acute dacryocystitis (clinical features and management).	412	414	J12(RS2), J17
7.	Dacryocystorhinostomy (DCR)—steps, complications, contraindications.	413	498	J10, J13, J15

CHAPTER 17 DISEASES OF ORBIT

Long Essay

1.	Orbital cellulites—etiology, clinical features and management.	426	393	D07(RS2), D08

Short Essays

1.	Proptosis—define, different causes (at age of 60 years), investigation and management.	420	388	D10(RS2), J08
2.	Discuss causes for uniocular proptosis.	421	388	D12(RS3)
3.	Orbital cellulitis—clinical features and management.	426	393	J11(RS2), J17(RS3), D17(RS3), J01, D04, J17
4.	Draw a neat labeled diagram of cavernous sinus and its connections.	428	24	D11
5.	Cavernous sinus thrombosis.	428	400	D07
6.	What is endocrine exophthalmos? Describe its mechanism and pathogenesis.	431	395	D02
7.	Describe eye manifestations of thyroid ophthalmopathy/clinical features of thyroid eye disease.	431	396	D07(RS2), D12, D14
8.	Blowout fracture (features).	440	450	D12(RS3), D09
9.	Name three destructive surgeries in ophthalmology and discuss about exenteration.	443	—	J08

Contd...

Contd...

	KHRN	BSAK	
Short Answers			
1. Orbital hemorrhage—mention three causes.	—	—	J03
2. Name the bones forming the medial wall of the orbit.	418	21	D10(RS2)
3. Proptosis (exophthalmos)—define, causes for (bilateral) proptosis (in adults/children).	420	388	J04, D09, J11, D11, J13, J15, J17
4. What is exophthalmus and enophthalmus? Mention two causes for each.	420, 424	388	D01
5. Mention causes for acute and gradual onset proptosis?	421	389	J02
6. Orbital cellulitis (features).	426	393	D15(RS3), D12
7. Lid signs in thyroid associated ophthalmopathy.	431	396	D11(RS2), J16(RS3), D09
8. Blowout fracture of orbit—state three signs.	440	450	D16(RS3)
9. What is exenteration? Name two indications for exenteration.	443	—	D10
CHAPTER 18 **OCULAR INJURIES**			
Long Essay			
1. Classify the various ocular injuries and describe effects of blunt injury over an eye.	444, 446	443	D11(RS2), J16(RS3), J09, D11
Short Essays			
1. Classification of ocular injures.	444	443	D16
2. Blunt ocular injury (mechanical effects, complications, management).	445	443	J12(RS2), D13(RS2), D05
3. Discuss the anterior segment features of blunt trauma to the eye.	447	445	J13
4. Traumatic hyphema.	447	445	J15(RS3)

Contd...

Contd...

		KHRN	BSAK	
5.	Describe the lens changes following blunt injury to the eye.	447	447	D01, J05, J15
6.	Traumatic cataract.	448	448	J10(RS2), D15
7.	Commotio retinae—define, treatment.	448	449	J13(RS3)
8.	Penetrating injury of the eye.	449	451	D18(RS3)
9.	Siderosis bulbi—etipathogenesis and clinical features.	452	456	J03, D14, D16
10.	Sympathetic ophthalmitis (clinical features, treatment).	455	239	J10(RS2), J11(RS2), D15(RS3), D17(RS3), D06, J07, J09, D13, D16
11.	Chemical injuries/alkali burns to the eye (grading, managements and complication).	456	459	J14(RS2), D16(RS3), J19(RS3), J05, D11, J14
Short Answers				
1.	Corneal foreign body—removal.	444	453	J18(RS3), D19(RS3)
2.	Enumerate the iris abnormalities following blunt trauma.	447	446	D12
3.	Iridodialysis.	447	446	D15
4.	What are the effects of blunt injury on the lens?	447	447	D08
5.	Rossette cataract.	448	448	J13(RS3)
6.	Berlin's edema.	448	449	J10(RS2)
7.	Enumerate complications of retained intraocular iron foreign body.	451	455	D07
8.	Chalcosis—define, eye manifestations.	452	457	J09(RS2), D10
9.	What is black eye and red eye? Mention three causes of red eye and one cause of black eye.	455	443	D02
10.	Sympathetic ophthalmitis (clinical features).	455	239	J08, D15

Contd...

Contd...

		KHRN	BSAK	
11.	Chemical injury/alkali burn to the eye—(late) complications.	458	459	D00, D13

Section IV: Ocular Therapeutics

CHAPTER 19 OCULAR PHARMACOLOGY

Short Essays

1.	Various methods of administration of drugs in ophthalmic diseases.	463	48	D15(RS3), J01, D01, D04
2.	Antiviral drugs in eye disorders.	466	50	J11(RS2), D17(RS3)
3.	Antifungal drugs.	468	51	J12(RS2)
4.	(Newer) antiglaucoma drugs—classify, one example for each, discuss in detail any one.	469	53	D07(RS2), J08(RS2), J15(RS3), D08
5.	Use of prostaglandins in ophthalmology.	469	308	J09(RS2)
6	Timolol maleate—mechanism of action, dose and side effects.	470	308	J06
7.	Pilocarpine—mode of action, uses and ocular complications.	472	309	D14(RS3), J17
8.	Corticosteroids in ophthalmology—indications (uses), contraindications and complications.	473	54	D09(RS2), D11(RS2), J16(RS3), J13
9.	Mention the uses of fluorescein in ophthalmology.	479	562	J08
10.	Cycloplegics.	593	52	D11(RS2), J16(RS3)
11.	Mydriatics, their actions and side effects.	593	52	J18(RS3)
12.	Atropine—uses in ophthalmology.	108, 164, 593	52	D07(RS2), D19(RS3)

Short Answers

1.	State three drugs given as intravitreal injection with its concentration and its indication.	464	49	D16(RS3)

Contd...

Contd...

		KHRN	BSAK	
2.	Mention three antiviral drugs?	466	50	D00
3.	Antifungal drugs.	468	51	D09(RS2)
4.	Classify antiglaucoma drugs.	469	53	D16
5.	Topical antiglacuoma drugs.	469	53	D15
6.	Mention three topical drugs and their mechanism of action in treatment of primary open angle glaucoma.	469	53	J14
7.	Mention three new antiglaucoma drugs and its dosage.	469	53	J08
8.	Name the drugs which decrease the aqueous production.	469	53	D10
9.	Timolol maleate (mode of action and side effects).	470	308	J13(RS3), D16(RS3), J18(RS3), D13
10.	Miotics.	471	51	J17(RS3), D03, J11
11.	Acetazolamide—three important side effects.	471	53	J05
12.	What are the pharmacological effects of pilocarpine in the eye? Mention its uses.	472	309	J07
13.	Mention three hyperosmotic agents and its dosage.	472	53	J10
14.	Steroid in ophthalmology (uses/three side effects).	473	54	J14(RS2), J03, J07, J11
15.	Mention six ocular diseases/three corneal ulcers in which steroid therapy is indicated.	474	54	D02, J17
16.	Uses of fluorescein in ophthalmology.	479	562	D13(RS2)
17.	Cycloplegic mydriatics in ophthalmology.	593	52	J08(RS2), J11(RS2), D13(RS2), D17(RS3), D18(RS3), J19(RS3)
18.	Mention three mydriatic agents with their duration of action.	593	52	D12(RS3), J06, D12

Contd...

Contd...

		KHRN	BSAK	
19.	Atropine sulphate (atropine eye drops)—three uses in ophthalmology.	108, 164, 593	52	D08(RS2), J15(RS3), D06

CHAPTER 20
LASERS AND CRYOTHERAPY IN OPHTHALMOLOGY

Short Essays

1.	What is Laser? Mention its (Nd-YAG laser) uses in ophthalmology.	481	558	J10, J15
2.	Lasers for posterior segment diseases in ophthalmology.	483	559	D15
3.	Uses of cryotherapy in ophthalmology	484	561	D18(RS3)

Short Answers

1.	Laser—define, types, three/six uses in ophthalmology.	481	558	D10(RS2), J19(RS3), D01, D03, J08, J09, D16
2.	YAG Laser.	482	558	J14(RS2)
3.	Mention the uses of lasers for anterior segment pathology.	483	559	D13
4.	Mention the uses of lasers in the management of retinal diseases.	483	559	D11
5.	Cryotherapy in ophthalmology—indications/three operations.	484	561	J09(RS2), D00

Section V: Systemic and Community Ophthalmology

CHAPTER 21
SYSTEMIC OPHTHALMOLOGY

Short Essays

1.	Vitamin A deficiency (xerophthalmia)—WHO classification, ocular manifestations, management.	487	511	D07(RS2), D09(RS2), D13(RS2), J18(RS3), D18(RS3), J03, J06, J10

Contd...

Contd...

	KHRN	BSAK	
2. Bitot's spot.	488	512	D14(RS3)
3. Mention the ocular manifestations of leprosy.	491	—	J08
Short Answers			
1. What are ocular components of myasthenia gravis.	—	—	J06
2. Vitamin A deficiency (WHO classification).	487	511	J12(RS2), J13(RS3)
3. Bitot's spots—clinical appearance, etiology and management (diet advised).	488	512	D10(RS2), D00
4. Give sources of vitamin A.	490	514	D05
5. AIDS—ocular manifestations/three important retinal lesions.	490	—	J10, D11, D15
6. What are the ocular manifestations of leprosy?	491	—	J14
CHAPTER 22 COMMUNITY OPHTHALMOLOGY			
Long Essay			
1. Discuss the National Program of Control of Blindness (NPCB) in detail.	502	504	D15
Short Essays			
1. Legal blindness.	496	502	D08(RS2)
2. Vision 2020.	499	515	D18(RS3), D14
3. National Trachoma Control Program.	501	508	J13(RS3)
4. What is trachoma control project?	501	508	D03
5. National Program for Control of Blindness—aims and objectives.	502	504	J02, J05
6. District Blindness Control Society (DBCS).	503	509	J19(RS3), D16
7. Eye bank—define, activities, methods of corneal preservation.	509	493	J01, D04, J12, J16, J17
8. Eye donation.	510	493	D00, D15
Short Answers			
1. Cause of permanent/incurable blindness.	—	—	D19(RS3), J01, D04

Contd...

Contd...

		KHRN	BSAK	
2.	Causes of preventable blindness.	496	503	J14(RS2), J03
3.	Legal, economic and social blindness—define, three causes.	496	502	J10(RS2), D10(RS2), J11(RS2), D17(RS3), D00, J12, D13, D16
4.	Vision 2020—objectives and diseases targeted.	499	515	D13(RS2), J15(RS3), D15(RS3), J17
5.	National Trachoma Control Program.	501	508	J10(RS2)
6.	National Programs for Control of Blindness—Objectives.	502	504	J11(RS2), D17(RS3), J06
7.	What are the three levels of National Program for Control of Blindness?	503	506	J07
8.	District Blindness Control Society.	503	509	D09(RS2)
9.	Childhood blindness (below three years)—causes.	506	505	D09(RS2), D11(RS2), J16(RS3), J07
10.	Eye bank—functions.	509	493	J02
11.	Eye donation.	510	493	J19(RS3)

Section VI: Practical Ophthalmology

CHAPTER 23 CLINICAL METHODS IN OPHTHALMOLOGY

Long Essays

1.	A 55-year-old man comes with painless progressive diminution of vision. Discuss the differential diagnosis.	514	264	D06
2.	Enumerate the causes for gradual loss of vision and discuss one cause in detail.	514	264	D12(RS3)
3.	Discuss the causes of sudden unilateral visual loss.	514	—	D09

Contd...

Contd...

		KHRN	BSAK	
Short Essays				
1.	Differential diagnosis of gradual loss of vision.	514	264	D19(RS3)
2.	Differential diagnosis of sudden loss of vision.	514	—	J14(RS2)
3.	A 20-year-old boy presents with history of floaters in his left eye. Discuss the causes and outline the management.	515, 268	—	D00
4.	What are the causes of papillary hypertrophy of conjunctiva? What is the difference between a follicle and a papilla in the conjunctiva?	521	147	D02
5.	Leukocoria (differential diagnosis).	526		J10(RS2), J06, D13
6.	Cherry red spot—causes.	529	333	J18(RS3), J10
7.	Tonometry—different techniques.	530	283	J19(RS3), D19(RS3)
8.	Classify tonometer. Mention briefly advantages and disadvantages of each.	530	119	J13(RS3)
9.	Describe the assessment and significance of visual field analysis.	532	303	D12
10.	B-scan—its uses in ophthalmology.	542	569	D15
Short Answers				
1.	What is Imbert-Fick principle?	—	285	D07(RS2)
2.	Sudden loss of vision—causes.	514	—	D18(RS3), J04, J10
3.	Gradual loss of vision—three causes.	514	—	J05
4.	Black spots in front of eyes—three causes.	515	—	D05
5.	Diplopia—causes.	515	—	J05, J16
6.	Colored halos—causes.	515	—	D14(RS3), J15(RS3), J17
7.	Snellen's chart and its applications.	516	103	D13(RS2)
8.	What is physiological role of blinking? What complications can absence blinking produce?	519	134	D02

Contd...

Contd...

		KHRN	BSAK	
9.	What are the causes of follicles in the conjunctiva?	520	147	D06, D07
10.	Mention three differences between papillary and follicular conjunctivitis.	520	147	J17
11.	Mention three importance differences between a conjunctival follicle and a papilla.	521	147	D11
12.	Decreased corneal sensation—causes.	523	111	D06
13.	Iris nodules—causes.	525	—	J17(RS3), J04, J06
14.	Define: (a) Polycoria, (b) Anisocoria, (c) Leukocoria.	525	219	D00
15.	Mydriasis—define, causes.	525	115	J02, D11, J16
16.	Name three pathological pupillary reactions.	526	44	J07
17.	Leukocoria (causes).	526	382	D14, D15, D16
18.	Cherry red spot—define, three causes.	529	333	D08(RS2), J12(RS2), J17(RS3), D01, J01, D04, D06, J13
19.	Soft exudates in retina—causes.	529	351	J04, D07
20.	Enumerate the various methods of recording intraocular pressure.	530	283	D00, J16
21.	Classify tonometers.	530	283	J09(RS2)
22.	Bitemporal hemianopia—define, two causes.	530	44	J03
23.	Give one cause and site of lesion for: (a) Bitemporal hemianopia, (b) Centro caecal scotoma, (c) Right sided homonymous hemianopia.	530	44, 364, 44	D00
24.	Mention the types of ultrasonogram used in ophthalmology. Name two indications for their use.	542	568	D11
25.	A-scan biometry.	542	568	D18(RS3)

Contd...

Contd...

	KHRN	BSAK	
CHAPTER 24 **CLINICAL OPHTHALMIC CASES**			
None			
CHAPTER 25 **DARKROOM PROCEDURES**			
Short Essays			
1. What is retinoscopy? Write briefly the principle of retinoscopy.	591	90	D11
2. Tabulate differences between direct and indirect ophthalmoscopy.	609	94	J09
Short Answers			
1. Gonioscopy (angle structures seen).	589	293	D15(RS3), J02, J16
2. Retinoscopy.	591	90	J14(RS2)
3. Enumerate methods to assess the corneal curvature.	596	575	D07
4. Pinhole test (principle).	599	549	D14(RS3), D18(RS3), D19(RS3), D10
5. Mention advantages and disadvantages between direct and indirect ophthalmoscopy.	609	94	J06
CHAPTER 26 **OPHTHALMIC INSTRUMENTS AND OPERATIVE OPHTHALMOLOGY**			
Short Essay			
1. Iridotomy.	632	487	J18(RS3)
Short Answers			
1. Enumerate types of anesthesia for intraocular surgery.	612	466	D18(RS3)
2. Mention six anesthetic complications of intraocular surgery.	629	466	D00

Contd...

Contd...

	KHRN	BSAK	
MISCELLANEOUS			
Long Essay			
1. Describe the various viral infections of the eye. How will you manage?	—	—	J10(RS2)
Short Essays			
1. Orbital apex syndrome.	—	—	J13(RS3)
2. Differential diagnosis of nodules near the limbus.	—	—	D09(RS2), D13(RS2)
3. Mention the causes of nodule at the limbus.	—	—	J14
4. Meibomian cell carcinoma.	—	143	D10(RS2)
Short Answers			
1. What is pseudohypopyon? Mention two conditions which cause pseudohypopyon.	—	114	J07, J16
2. Mention three ophthalmic manifestations of pituitary tumors.	—	—	J07
3. Mention three conditions where circumciliary congestion is seen.	—	146	J08
4. What is Hutchinson's triad?	—	—	D08
5. Six causes of nodule at limbus.	—	—	D10(RS2), J17

3

Otorhinolaryngology

REFERENCES

1. PL Dhingra, Shruti Dhingra **(DNGR)**: Diseases of Ear, Nose and Throat, 7th Edition, Elsevier Medical Science, New Delhi, ₹ 1345/-
2. Mohan Bansal **(BNSL)**: Essentials of Ear, Nose and Throat, 1st Edition, Jaypee Brothers Medical Publishers (P) Ltd., New Delhi, ₹ 895/-

COURSE CONTENTS

DISEASES OF THE EAR

- Surgical anatomy
  - External, middle and inner ear
- Physiology of hearing and vestibular function
- Examination of the ear
  - Tuning fork tests, hearing assessment in children—broad outline, referred pain in the ear, otalgia, tinnitus
- Deafness
  - Types and causes
- Diseases of external ear
  - Perichondritis, otitis externa, cerumen, foreign body, furunculosis, keratosis
- Diseases of middle ear
  - Acute and chronic suppurative otitis media, obturans, otitis media with effusion, otosclerosis, cholesteatoma
- Audiometry
  - Pure tone
- Functional examination of inner ear (vestibule)
  - Calorie test, positional nystagmus test
- Deaf mutism
- Meniere's disease
- Complications of otitis media
  - Mastoiditis (acute and chronic), lateral sinus thrombosis, labyrinthltis, otogenic brain abscess
- Mastoidectomy
  - Principles
- Tumors of the ear
  - Glomus, acoustic neuroma.

DISEASES OF THE NOSE AND PARANASAL SINUSES

- Surgical anatomy and physiology of nose and paranasal sinuses including olfaction
- Congenital diseases of the nose, cleft lip and palate and choanal atresia
- Diseases of external nose
  - Furunculosis, vestibulitis, rhinophyma, rodent ulcer
- Trauma to nose and paranasal sinus
  - Fracture of nasal bones, blowout fracture of orbit, fracture of maxilla with Le Fort classification
- Foreign body in nose
  - Classification of foreign bodies and management of animate and inanimate foreign bodies, rhinolith
- Causes of epistaxis and management
- Disease of nasal septum
  - Hematoma, abscess, derived nasal septum (DNS), perforation

- Diseases of nasal cavity
  - Acute rhinitis, nasal diphtheria, granulomatous conditions of the nose, allergic rhinitis, vasomotor rhinitis, atrophic rhinitis, fungal infections of nose and paranasal sinuses
- Diseases of paranasal sinuses
  - Acute and chronic sinusitis, complications of sinusitis and management
- Sinonasal polyposis
  - Diagnosis and management
- Basic principles of Functional endoscopic sinus surgery (FESS)
- Tumors of the nose and paranasal sinuses
  - Benign tumors like papilloma, inverted papilloma, fibrous dysplasia
  - Malignant tumors like squamous cell carcinoma, melanoma, olfactory neuroblastoma.

DISEASES OF THE NASOPHARYNX

- Surgical anatomy and physiology of nasopharynx
- Nasopharyngeal carcinoma
  - Diagnosis and management
- Adenoid
  - Diagnosis and management
- Juvenile angiofibroma
  - Diagnosis and management.

DISEASES OF THE PHARYNX

- Surgical anatomy and physiology of oral cavity, oropharynx, tonsil, Waldeyer's ring
- Anatomy of retropharyngeal and parapharyngeal spaces
- Physiology of mastication
- Diseases of the tonsils
  - Acute and chronic tonsillitis
    - Diagnosis and management
  - Vincent's angina
    - Diagnosis and management
  - Diphtheritic tonsillitis
    - Diagnosis and management
- Neck space infections and abscess
  - Retropharyngeal abscess, parapharyngeal abscess, peritonsillar abscess, Ludwig's angina
- Surgical anatomy and physiology of salivary glands, submandibular sialadenitis, salivary calculi, parotitis, tumors of salivary glands.

DISEASES OF THE LARYNX

- Surgical anatomy and physiology of larynx with reference to phonation and respiration

- Acute infection of larynx
  - Acute laryngitis, laryngotracheobronchitis (LTB), diphtheritic laryngitis, acute epiglottitis
- Stridor
  - Causes of stridor and management
- Hoarseness of voice
  - History taking, causes, management
- Chronic infections of larynx
  - Chronic nonspecific and specific laryngitis, granulomatous conditions of larynx
- Neurological infections of larynx
  - Cord palsy
    - Diagnosis and management
- Tumors of larynx
  - Diagnosis of laryngeal tumors and management.

DISEASES OF THE TRACHEA

- Surgical anatomy of trachea, stridor, tracheostomy in detail.

DISEASES OF THE ESOPHAGUS

- Surgical anatomy, physiology of deglutition
- Causes of dysphagia, diagnosis and management
- Diseases such as congenital atresia, injuries (traumatic and chemical)
- Foreign body
- Esophagoscopy
- Neurological problems
- Oncology.

DISEASES OF THE BRONCHUS

- Bronchoscopy
  - Indications, contraindications and complications of foreign body in bronchus.

UNIVERSITY EXAMINATION PATTERN

Eligibility for Writing the University Examination

The candidate should have at least 35% aggregate in the two of the three internals conducted by the college and should also have minimum 75% attendance in Theory and Practical classes conducted.

Criteria for Passing the University Examination

The candidate should secure minimum 50% in the university theory examination (University theory + Viva voce) and the university practical examinations separately. Internal assessment marks would not be considered for passing criteria, however, they would be added to final marks to determine class of passing.

Distribution of Marks

	Internal Assessment		*University Examination*	
	Maximum marks	*Minimum marks to qualify*	*Maximum marks*	*Minimum marks to pass*
Theory examination	30 marks	11 marks	100 marks	60 marks
Viva-voce	—	—	20 marks	
Practical examination	20 marks	07 marks	80 marks	40 marks

Distribution of Marks for University Examination

Theory Examination

It is of 150 marks in total, which consist of:

University Examination	100 marks
University Viva Voce	20 marks
Theory Internals	30 marks

Clinical Examination

It is of 100 marks in total, which consists of:

University Clinical	80 marks
Clinical Internals	20 marks

Theory Examination

There shall be one theory paper carrying 100 marks. The pattern of questions would be of three types.

2 Long Essay Questions	2 × 10 marks	20 marks
10 Short Essay Questions	10 × 5 marks	50 marks
10 Short Answer Questions	10 × 3 marks	30 marks
	Total	**100 marks**

Clinical Examination

Practical examination will carry 80 marks (2 cases of 40 marks each).

Viva Voce Examination

Viva voce carries 20 marks.

Instruments + viva	10 marks
X-rays + viva	10 marks

Question Bank

	DNGR	BNSL	

Section I: Diseases of Ear

CHAPTER 1
ANATOMY OF EAR

Long Essay

1. Describe briefly the anatomy of the middle ear cleft with a suitable labeled diagram.	5	7	J12(RS2), D18(RS3)

Short Essays

1. Describe the normal tympanic membrane. Draw neat labeled diagram (of right side).	3	6	J04, J06, J12
2. Anatomy of the middle ear cleft with diagram.	5	7	J11(RS2), D15(RS3), D16(RS3), J19(RS3), D05, J14
3. Surgical anatomy of medial wall of the middle ear (draw a labeled diagram).	6	9	J08
4. Middle ear contents and their functions.	9	10	D07(RS2)

Short Answers

1. Pinna—nerve supply.	3	4	J12, D13
2. Tympanic membrane—anatomy/ labeled diagram (left/right).	3	6	J16(RS3), J10, D10
3. Nerve supply of external auditory canal (external ear).	5	6	D11(RS2), J19(RS3), D08, J13
4. Middle ear cleft and its contents.	5	7	J02, J17
5. Draw labeled diagram of medial wall of middle ear.	7	10	D07
6. MacEwen's triangle.	7	12	D13(RS2), D14(RS3), J19(RS3), D13, J14, J16
7. Enumerate the cells of the mastoid air cell system.	7	13	D12
8. Intratympanic muscles (nerve supply).	9	11	J15(RS3)

Contd...

Contd...

		DNGR	BNSL	
9.	Stapedius muscle.	9	11	J12
10.	Tympanic plexus.	9	11	D09(RS2), J11, D14
CHAPTER 2 PERIPHERAL RECEPTORS AND PHYSIOLOGY OF AUDITORY AND VESTIBULAR SYSTEM				
Long Essay				
1.	Describe the physiology and mechanism of hearing.	15	24	D07(RS2)
Short Essays				
1.	Theories of hearing.	—	—	J11(RS2), D16(RS3)
2.	Organ of Corti.	15	16	J12(RS2), J13(RS3)
3.	Physiology of hearing.	15	24	D15
4.	Middle ear—impedance matching mechanism/transformer mechanism.	16	25	J15(RS3), J06, D13
5.	Role of cochlea in hearing.	17	17	D05
6.	Physiology of equilibrium.	20	28	D16
Short Answers				
1.	Discuss the theories of hearing.	—	—	J14(RS2)
2.	Otoliths.	18	—	D14
CHAPTER 3 AUDIOLOGY AND ACOUSTICS				
Short Answer				
1.	Decibel.	21	39	D08
CHAPTER 4 ASSESSMENT OF HEARING				
Short Essays				
1.	How to assess a patient of hearing loss in outpatient department?	23	40	J10
2.	Tuning fork tests and their significance.	23	41	J19(RS3), D07, J08, D08, D14

Contd...

OTORHINOLARYNGOLOGY

Contd...

		DNGR	BNSL	
3.	Rinne's test.	24	41	J10(RS2)
4.	Pure tone audiometry (pure tone audiogram).	25	43	D11(RS2), J18(RS3), J16
5.	Tympanometry.	26	46	D08(RS2), D18(RS3), D15
6.	Brainstem evoked response audiometry (BERA).	29	48	D08(RS2)
7.	Otoacoustic emissions.	29	49	J14(RS2)
Short Answers				
1.	Tuning fork tests.	23	41	D07(RS2)
2.	Rinne's test and its clinical significance.	24	41	D10(RS2), J11(RS2), D12(RS3), D16(RS3), D00, D03, J04, D04, J10
3.	False-negative Rinne's test.	24	42	J14
4.	Weber's test.	24	42	D14(RS3), J15(RS3), D19(RS3), D05, D02, D06, D13
5.	Absolute bone conduction test.	24	43	J02, J16
6.	Schwabach's test.	24	43	J16(RS3)
7.	Bing's test.	24	43	J10(RS2)
8.	Pure tone audiometry.	25	43	J09
9.	Speech audiometry.	25	45	J09(RS2)
10.	Tympanograms.	27	46	J18(RS3)
11.	Acoustic reflex tests.	27	47	J17(RS3)

OTORHINOLARYNGOLOGY

CHAPTER 5
HEARING LOSS

Long Essay

1.	Discuss sound conducting mechanism in brief. Discuss the cause and principles of management of conductive hearing loss.	16, 31	24, 51	J08

Contd...

Contd...

	DNGR	BNSL	
Short Essays			
1. Treatment of bilateral profound hearing loss.	—	—	D03
2. Classify hearing loss and enumerate the causes of conductive hearing loss.	31	51	J15
3. Conductive deafness (causes).	31	51	D08(RS2), D00, J01, D04
4. Tympanoplasty (classification).	31	438	D08, J11, D16
5. Sensorineural (SN) deafness—causes.	34	59	J03
6. Ototoxicity (ototoxic drugs and management).	35	61	D08(RS2), D17(RS3), D00, D02, D04, D14, J16, J17
7. Noise-induced hearing loss.	36	63	D09(RS2), J13
8. Sudden SN hearing loss—causes and management.	38	64	D15(RS3), J17(RS3)
9. Sudden hearing loss (causes).	38	64	J05
10. Presbyacusis (senile deafness)—management.	39	65	J14(RS2), J07, D10, J15
11. Unilateral sensorineural deafness.	41	59	D12
Short Answers			
1. Discuss prerequisite for successful type I tympanoplasty.	31	—	D07
2. Ototoxicity—prevention and management.	35	61	J16(RS3), D05, D06
3. Acoustic trauma.	36	63	J12(RS2), J13(RS3)
4. Sudden hearing loss.	38	64	J16(RS3)
5. Malingering.	39	67	J07

Contd...

Contd...

	DNGR	BNSL	
CHAPTER 6 **ASSESSMENT OF VESTIBULAR FUNCTIONS**			
Short Essays			
1. Vestibular function tests.	43	131	J09(RS2), D09(RS2)
2. Fistula test and its significance.	43	131	J09
Short Answers			
1. Labrynthine nystagmus.	43	130	D15
2. Fistula test.	43	131	D13(RS2), D15(RS3), D17(RS3), D08, J11, D12
3. Hennebert's sign.	43	131	J10(RS2)
4. Romberg's test.	43	134	J12
5. Calorie test and its significance.	45	133	J17(RS3), J01, J04, J07
CHAPTER 7 **DISORDERS OF VESTIBULAR SYSTEM**			
Short Essays			
1. Evaluation of vertigo in a 60-year-old female.	—	130	J13
2. Causes (aural) of vertigo.	47	136	J11, D16
3. Vesitubular neuronitis.	47	137	D10(RS2)
Short Answer			
1. Benign paroxysmal positional vertigo—management.	47	136	D15(RS3), J17(RS3)
CHAPTER 8 **DISEASES OF EXTERNAL EAR**			
Long Essay			
1. Draw a labeled diagram of middle ear cleft. Discuss the etiopathology, symptomatology and management of malignant otitis externa.	6, 55	7, 92	D03, J16

Contd...

Contd...

	DNGR	BNSL	
Short Essays			
1. Auricular hematoma (cauliflower ear).	52	86	D11, J12
2. Perichondritis of the pinna.	53	86	J19(RS3)
3. Otitis externa.	54	89	D16
4. Otomycosis.	55	90	J09(RS2), D19(RS3), D02, D07, J10, J12, D15
5. Malignant otitis externa (etiology, clinical features and management).	55	92	D10(RS2), J17(RS3), D17(RS3), D18(RS3), J02, D06, J09, D11, D13, J14
6. Aural syringing—indications, contraindication, procedure and complications.	56	91	J04, J08
7. Foreign body in external auditory canal—types, causes and management.	57	88	D03, J10
8. Keratosis obturans.	58	90	J02, D05, D11, D12, J16, J17
9. Traumatic perforation of the ear (tympanic membrane)—treatment.	59	94	J19(RS3), D03
Short Answers			
1. Hematoma auris (management).	52	86	J06, D06
2. Otitis externa.	54	89	D08(RS2), D12(RS3), D13(RS2), J16(RS3), J13
3. Otomycosis (organisms causing/ management).	55	90	D11(RS2), J17(RS3), J04, J06, J07, D10
4. Malignant otitis externa.	55	92	J10(RS2), J04, D08
5. Cerumen (wax)—management.	56	91	J01, J03, D06

Contd...

Contd...

	DNGR	BNSL	
6. Aural syringing—indications.	56	—	J14
7. Foreign bodies in the ear.	57	88	J08(RS2)
8. Keratosis obturans.	58	90	J08(RS2), J12(RS2), J13(RS3), D07, J15
9. Traumatic perforation of tympanic membrane.	59	93	D09(RS2)
10. Tympanosclerosis.	59	93	D05, D13
CHAPTER 9 EUSTACHIAN TUBE AND ITS DISORDERS			
Short Essays			
1. Eustachian tube.	61	95	D16
2. Eustachian tube patency tests.	62	97	J10(RS2)
Short Answers			
1. Eustachian tube.	61	95	D09(RS2)
2. Valsalva maneuver.	62	98	D05
CHAPTER 10 DISORDERS OF MIDDLE EAR			
Long Essays			
1. Acute suppurative otitis media—etiology, pathology, symptoms, signs, diagnosis and treatment.	67	101	D12(RS3), J15(RS3), J16(RS3), J19(RS3), D07, D08
2. Enumerate the causes of conductive hearing loss with intact tympanic membrane. Describe the etiology, clinical features and management of serous otitis media (secretory otitis media/otitis media with effusion in a 4-year-old child).	32, 69	52, 106	J06, J15
3. Nonsuppurative otitis media—etiology, pathology, clinical features, investigations and management.	71	105	J17

Contd...

Contd...

	DNGR	BNSL	
Short Essays			
1. Acute suppurative otitis media—treatment (surgical).	67	101	J18(RS3), D18(RS3), D03
2. Secretory otitis media/otitis media with effusion/Glue ear—management.	69	105	D13(RS2), D01, D02, J05, J10, D10, J10, J11
Short Answer			
1. Secretory otitis media/glue ear—treatment.	69	105	D17(RS3), J01, J04
CHAPTER 11 CHOLESTEATOMA AND CHRONIC SUPPURATIVE OTITIS MEDIA			
Long Essays			
1. Define cholesteatoma. Describe its classification, etiopathogenesis, clinical features and management of cholesteatoma.	73	110	J13(RS3), J17(RS3), J10, D13
2. Enumerate the common causes of conductive deafness. Discuss in detail the etiology, pathology, clinical features and management of tubotympanic type of chronic suppurative otitis media.	32, 75	114	D11(RS2), J07
3. What is cholesteatoma? Describe the etiology, pathology, clinical features and management of atticoantral type of chronic suppurative otitis media. Discuss briefly the complications of atticoantral disease.	73, 78, 83	110	D13(RS2), D01, J05, D14
Short Essays			
1. Cholesteatoma—etiopathogenesis (theories of formation of cholesteatoma), management.	73	110	D07(RS2), D10(RS2), D14(RS3), J18(RS3), J11, D14
2. Draw neat labeled diagrams showing different types of perforations of the tympanic membrane.	77	110	D06

Contd...

Contd...

	DNGR	BNSL	
Short Answers			
1. What is cholesteatoma? Mention in brief about theories of its formation.	73	110	D07, D16
2. Classify cholesteatoma.	74	111	D02, J04
3. Perforation in pars tensa (types and clinical significance).	76	109	D01, D10, D15

CHAPTER 12
COMPLICATIONS OF OTITIS MEDIA

Long Essays			
1. Enumerate the complications of otitis media. Discuss the management of atticoantral type of chronic suppurative otitis media (CSOM).	83, 80	118, 113	D12
2. Give an account of complications of CSOM and name the warning signs to detect such complications in a case of CSOM.	83	118	D11
3. Enumerate extracranial complications of chronic suppurative otitis media. Discuss any one in detail.	83	118	J09
4. Classify and enumerate the complications of suppurative otitis media. Discuss the clinical features and management of lateral sinus thrombophlebitis.	83, 92	118, 126	J04, D06
5. Discuss the etiopathology, clinical features, complications and management of acute (coalescent) mastoiditis.	84	118	J11(RS2), D15(RS3), D16(RS3), J13, J14
Short Essays			
1. Extratemporal complications of chronic suppurative otitis media.	—	120	D08(RS2)
2. Complication of CSOM.	83	118	J18(RS3), J14
3. Sequel of otitis media.	84	117	D19(RS3)
4. Intratemporal complications of CSOM.	84	118	D09(RS2)
5. Acute coalescent mastoiditis (signs and symptoms).	84	118	D12(RS3), J03, D15, J16

Contd...

Contd...

		DNGR	BNSL	
6.	Outline differences of acute mastoiditis with furuncle of external auditory canal (EAC).	86	120	D08
7.	Acute mastoid abscess.	86	120	D10(RS2), J19(RS3)
8.	Differential diagnosis of post-aural. abscess.	86	121	J08(RS2)
9.	Gradenigo's syndrome.	88	121	J12(RS2), J13(RS3)
10.	Lateral sinus thrombosis.	92	126	J09(RS2)

Short Answers

1.	Mention extracranial complications of CSOM.	83	118	J01
2.	List intracranial complications of CSOM.	84	118	J03
3.	Pathology of surgical mastoiditis.	84	119	D03
4.	Furunculosis of ear.	86	120	D15
5.	Bezold's abscess.	87	121	J12(RS2), J13(RS3)
6.	Gradenigo's syndrome.	88	121	D09(RS2), D00, D04, J07
7.	Lateral sinus thrombosis.	92	126	D07(RS2)
8.	Griensinger's sign.	93	127	J11, D11
9.	Otitic hydrocephalus.	93	127	D13

CHAPTER 13
OTOSCLEROSIS

Long Essay

1.	Enumerate the causes of conductive deafness in a 15-year-old girl. Describe the etiology, pathology, clinical features, investigations and management of otosclerosis.	32, 95	52	D10(RS2), J14(RS2), J18(RS3), D19(RS3), J01, D02, J12, J16, D16

Short Essays

1.	Otosclerosis (otospongiosis)—define, investigations, management (surgical treatment).	95	52	D09(RS2), D14(RS3), D06
2.	Carhart's notch.	96	55	D16

Contd...

Contd...

	DNGR	BNSL	
Short Answers			
1. What is otosclerosis? What are its signs and symptoms?	95	52	D18(RS3)
2. Paracusis Willisii.	96	55	D15(RS3)
3. Schwartz's sign.	96	55	J11
4. Carhart's notch.	96	55	D11(RS2)
5. Management of otosclerosis.	97	55	J13

CHAPTER 14

FACIAL NERVE AND ITS DISORDERS

Short Essays			
1. Intratemporal course of facial nerve.	99	149	D08(RS2)
2. Otological causes for facial paralysis.	103	154	D08(RS2), J11(RS2), D16(RS3)
3. Bell's palsy (etiology and treatment).	103	154	D12(RS3), J18(RS3), D18(RS3), J01, J11
4. Herpes zoster oticus (Ramsay-Hunt syndrome).	105	156	J09(RS2), J15, J17
5. Topodiagnostic tests for facial nerve palsy.	107	153	D10(RS2)
Short Answers			
1. Middle ear causes of facial nerve paralysis.	103	154	J05
2. Bell's palsy (etiology/management).	103	154	J14(RS2), D13
3. Ramsay-Hunt syndrome (herpes zoster oticus).	105	156	D17(RS3), D19(RS3), J03
4. Schirmer's test.	107	153	J17
5. Crocodile tears.	108	154	J09

Contd...

Contd...

	DNGR	BNSL	
CHAPTER 15 **MENIERE'S DISEASE**			
Long Essay			
1. Meniere's disease—etiopathogenesis, symptoms, signs, investigations and management.	111	138	D08(RS2), J10(RS2), D17(RS3), D00, D05
Short Essay			
1. Meniere's disease (clinical features and management).	111	138	J11(RS2), D12(RS3), J16(RS3), D16(RS3), J05, D07, J13
Short Answers			
1. Lermoyez syndrome.	114	139	J15
2. Treatment (acute attack) of Meniere's disease.	114	140	J03, J09
CHAPTER 16 **TUMORS OF EXTERNAL EAR**			
Short Essay			
1. Preauricular sinus.	117	86	D17(RS3)
Short Answers			
1. Preauricular sinus.	117		D18(RS3), D12, J15
2. Exostosis in external auditory canal.	118	160	J11(RS2), D16(RS3)
CHAPTER 17 **TUMORS OF MIDDLE EAR AND MASTOID**			
Short Essay			
1. Glomus tumor (tympanicus)—clinical features.	121	162	D13(RS2), J15
Short Answer			
1. Glomus tympanicum.	121	162	J08(RS2)

Contd...

Contd...

	DNGR	BNSL	
CHAPTER 18 **ACOUSTIC NEUROMA**			
Short Essay			
1. Clinical features of acoustic neuroma.	125	166	D11(RS2)
Short Answers			
1. Vestibular Schwanoma—clinical features.	125	166	J09(RS2)
2. Hitselberger's sign.	125	166	D11
CHAPTER 19 **THE DEAF CHILD**			
Short Essay			
1. Deaf child (causes, investigations—auditory tests).	129	69	D08(RS2), J16(RS3), D01, J05, J06, J14
CHAPTER 20 **REHABILITATION OF THE HEARING IMPAIRED**			
Short Essays			
1. Hearing rehabilitation of deaf child.	135	74	J11
2. Hearing aids.	135	76	D11(RS2), D14(RS3)
3. Cochlear implants.	138	81	J12(RS2), J13(RS3)
Short Answers			
1. Hearing aid.	135	76	J09(RS2), D13(RS2), J04, J07
2. Bone anchored hearing aids.	136	79	J15(RS3)
3. Cochlear implant.	138	81	D08(RS2), J02
CHAPTER 21 **OTALGIA (EARACHE)**			
Long Essay			
1. Acute earache—causes and management.	143	32	D10

Contd...

Contd...

	DNGR	BNSL	
Short Essay			
1. Referred otalgia.	143	33	J10(RS2), D15(RS3), J16
Short Answers			
1. Acute otalgia.	143	32	D15
2. Causes of pain in the ear.	143	33	D02, J03
3. Referred otalgia (three causes).	143	33	D08(RS2), D18(RS3), J16
CHAPTER 22 TINNITUS			
Short Essay			
1. Tinnitus—define, classification, causes.	145	35	J15(RS3), J02, J03, D08
Short Answer			
1. Tinnitus.	145	35	D12(RS3)
Section II: Diseases of Nose and Paranasal Sinuses			
CHAPTER 23 ANATOMY OF NOSE			
Short Essays			
1. Anatomy of lateral wall of the nose (labeled diagram).	149	171	D07(RS2), D14(RS3), D07, J09, J11
2. Osteomeatal complex.	150	173	D09(RS2), D11(RS2), D18(RS3)
3. Arterial and nerve supply of lateral wall of nose.	197, 153	174	J16
Short Answers			
1. Anatomy of middle meatus of nose.	150	173	J05
2. Osteomeatal complex.	150	173	J12(RS2), J13(RS3), J18(RS3), D02, J03, J12, J17

Contd...

Contd...

	DNGR	BNSL	
CHAPTER 24 **PHYSIOLOGY OF NOSE**			
Short Essays			
1. Olfactory area.	—	—	J12(RS2), J13(RS3)
2. Physiology of nose and paranasal sinus (PNS).	157	179	D15(RS3)
3. Mucociliary blanket of nose.	157	180	D17(RS3)
Short Answers			
1. Olfactory area.	—	—	D17(RS3)
2. Functions of the nasal cavities and paranasal sinuses.	157, 211	179, 182	J06, D06, D07, J12
3. Mucociliary blanket.	157	180	D19(RS3)
4. Mucocilliary mechanism.	157	180	D00, D04
5. Anosmia.	159	187	D14(RS3)
CHAPTER 25 **DISEASES OF EXTERNAL NOSE AND NASAL VESTIBULE**			
Short Essays			
1. Describe the etiology, pathology and management of saddle nose.	161	197	D01, D02
2. Rhinophyma (potato nose).	162	198	D11
3. Treatment of furunculosis.	163	196	D03
Short Answers			
1. Saddle nose (treatment).	161	197	D14(RS3), J15
2. Rhinophyma.	162	198	J11(RS2), D13(RS2), D16(RS3), J14
3. Nasal furuncle.	163	196	J15(RS3), J19(RS3)
4. Vestibulitis of nose.	163	196	D12(RS3), D13(RS2), J12

Contd...

Contd...

	DNGR	BNSL	
CHAPTER 26			
NASAL SEPTUM AND ITS DISEASES			
Long Essay			
1. Discuss etiology, types, clinical features and management of deviated nasal septum.	165	230	J08, D12
Short Essays			
1. Describe the anatomy of nasal septum. Discuss septal surgeries.	165, 471	172, 447	J17(RS3)
2. Deviated nasal septum—types, causes and treatment.	165	230	J14(RS2), D18(RS3)
3. Nasal septal hematoma.	168	231	J12
4. Septal abscess.	168	232	D15(RS3)
5. Septal perforation (clinical features and management).	169	232	J11(RS2), D16(RS3), J07
Short Answers			
1. Anatomy of the nasal septum (bones taking part in the formation/labeled diagram).	165	172	D08, J15
2. Chevallet fracture.	165	230	D16
3. Jarjavay fracture.	165	229	J10(RS2)
4. Hematoma septum (management).	168	231	D17(RS3), D00, D01, D04, J05, D05, D14
5. Septal abscess (management).	168	232	D12(RS3), D02, J11, D13
6. Nasal septal perforation (causes/ treatment).	169	232	D07(RS2), D11(RS2), J17(RS3), J06, D12
CHAPTER 27			
ACUTE AND CHRONIC RHINITIS			
Long Essay			
1. Atrophic rhinitis—etiology, pathology, clinical features, investigations and management.	172	214	D14(RS3), D19(RS3), J03, J09, D10, J13, J15

Contd...

Contd...

	DNGR	BNSL	
Short Essays			
1. Atrophic rhinitis (causes, clinical features and management/surgical treatment).	172	214	D13(RS2), J14(RS2), D15(RS3), D18(RS3), D00, J01, D02, D04, D07, D12, J14, J17
2. Rhinitis sicca.	174	216	J11(RS2), D16(RS3)
3. Rhinitis caseosa.	174	216	D12(RS3), J07, D14
CHAPTER 28 GRANULOMATOUS DISEASES OF NOSE			
Long Essay			
1. What is rhinosporidiosis? Describe its pathology, clinical features and treatment.	177	218	D07
Short Essays			
1. Rhinoscleroma (etiology, stages, clinical features, investigations and management).	175	216	D13(RS2), J14(RS2), D19(RS3), J07, D07, J09, D10, D12
2. Fungal infections of nose and paranasal sinuses.	177	218	J05
3. Nasal rhinosporidiosis (etiology, clinical features and management).	177	218	J10(RS2), D13(RS2), D01, J02, D06, D11
4. Mucormycosis of nose and paranasal sinuses.	178	218	J09(RS2), D02
5. Midline granuloma.	—	—	J09(RS2)
Short Answers			
1. Non healing midline granuloma.	—	—	J15(RS3)

Contd...

Contd...

		DNGR	BNSL	
2.	Rhinoscleroma—pathology.	175	216	D07(RS2), J16(RS3), J04, J08
3.	Rhinosporidiosis—histopathology/ management.	177	218	J17(RS3), J18(RS3), D03

CHAPTER 29
MISCELLANEOUS DISORDERS OF NASAL CAVITY

Short Essays

1.	Nasal foreign body.	181	244	D10
2.	Rhinolith—etiology, clinical features and management.	181	244	J01, D01, J12
3.	Nasal myiasis.	181	245	D13
4.	Choanal atresia.	183	233	D13(RS2)
5.	Cerebrospinal fluid rhinorrhea (etiology, clinical features and management).	183	242	J10(RS2), D12(RS3), D14(RS3), J18(RS3), D19(RS3), J03, J16

Short Answers

1.	Rhinolith.	181	244	D08(RS2), J12(RS2), J13(RS3), J17(RS3), D18(RS3), J07, J09, J15
2.	Nasal myiasis (management).	181	245	D07(RS2), J12(RS2), J14(RS2), J01, D07, J11
3.	Choanal atresia.	183	233	J08(RS2), D08(RS2), J12, D14
4.	Cerebrospinal fluid (CSF) rhinorrhea.	183	242	D03

Contd...

Contd...

	DNGR	BNSL	
CHAPTER 30 **ALLERGIC RHINITIS**			
Long Essay			
1. Allergic rhinitis—etiology, clinical features, investigations and treatment.	187	222	J12
Short Essays			
1. Pathophysiology of nasal allergy.	187	222	D09(RS2)
2. Allergic rhinitis (clinical features, management).	187	222	J02, D05, J11, J16
Short Answers			
1. Allergic rhinitis.	187	222	D03
2. Tests to screen nasal allergies.	188	224	D15, D16
3. Management of allergic rhinitis.	189	224	J18(RS3), D01
CHAPTER 31 **VASOMOTOR AND OTHER FORMS OF NONALLERGIC RHINITIS**			
Short Essay			
1. Describe vasomotor rhinitis (etiology, clinical features, management).	191	226	J12(RS2), J13(RS3), J16(RS3), J19(RS3), D00, D04
Short Answers			
1. Vasomotor rhinitis.	191	226	J09(RS2)
2. Rhinitis medicamentosa.	191	227	J09(RS2), D10(RS2), J14(RS2), D02, J04, D11, J13, J16, J17
CHAPTER 32 **NASAL POLYP**			
Long Essays			
1. Describe the anatomy of the lateral wall of the nasal cavity with management of nasal polyposis.	149, 196	171, 211	D13

Contd...

Contd...

		DNGR	BNSL	
2.	Describe the etiology, clinical features and management of nasal polyposis.	193	209	D13(RS2), J11
3.	Enumerate the differential diagnosis of unilateral nasal mass. Discuss the etiopathology, clinical features, investigations and management of ethmoidal polyposis.	194, 193	188, 209	J10(RS2), D12(RS3), D17(RS3), J06, D06, D15
Short Essays				
1.	Sinonasal polyposis (etiology and management).	193	209	J15(RS3), J17(RS3)
2.	Antrochoanal polyp (Killian's polyp)—clinical features, treatment.	193	210	D08, J10, D11, J17
3.	Unilateral nasal obstruction—causes/ differential diagnosis.	194	188	J06, D08, J10
4.	Bilateral nasal obstruction—differential diagnosis.	194	188	D03
5.	Differences between ethmoidal and antrochoanal polyp.	195	210	J16(RS3), D03, D07, J09
Short Answers				
1.	Nasal polyp.	193	209	J16(RS3)
2.	Antrochoanal polyp.	193	210	J04
3.	Ethmoidal polyp.	193	209	D03
4.	Young's syndrome.	194	209	D11
5.	Causes of nasal obstruction.	194	188	D15
6	Causes of unilateral nasal obstruction (mention six).	194	188	D19(RS3), J17
7.	Differences between ethmoidal polyp and antro choanal polyp.	195	210	D10(RS2)

CHAPTER 33
EPISTAXIS

Long Essay

1.	Describe the etiology, pathology, clinical features, investigations and management of epistaxis (in a 16-year-old boy/40-year-old man/60-year-old man).	197	190	J09(RS2), D11(RS2), J12(RS2), J13(RS3), J14(RS2), J02, J04, J05, D11, J14

Contd...

Contd...

	DNGR	BNSL	
Short Essays			
1. Blood supply of nose.	197	174	J15(RS3)
2. Discuss about Little's area with diagram and its clinical importance.	197	174	D10, D15
3. Epistaxis (investigations/management).	197	190	D16
Short Answers			
1. Blood supply of nasal septum.	197	174	D17(RS3)
2. Little's area (Kiesselbach's plexus).	197	174	J11(RS2), J13(RS3), D13(RS2), D16(RS3), D19(RS3), J01, D05, J07, J08, D08, J11, D12, J13, D16
3. Posterior epistaxis.	199	191	J08(RS2)
4. Management of acute epistaxis.	199	192	J10
5. First aid measures for epistaxis.	199	192	J06, D06
6. Anterior nasal packing.	200	192	J10(RS2)
7. Postnasal packing.	200	193	J08(RS2), D12
CHAPTER 34			
TRAUMA TO THE FACE			
Short Essays			
1. Fractures of middle third of face.	203	237	D10(RS2)
2. Nasal bone fractures—types, causes, management.	203	237	D12(RS3), D17(RS3), J18(RS3), D03, D06, J17
3. Tripod fracture.	205	239	J15
4. Blowout fracture of orbit.	206	239	D07(RS2)
5. Le Fort fractures of maxilla.	207	240	D09(RS2), J11(RS2), D16(RS3), J10

Contd...

Contd...

	DNGR	BNSL	
6. Le Fort II fracture.	207	240	J13
7. Oroantral fistula.	208	242	D14
Short Answers			
1. Fracture of nasal bone (nasal bone fractures).	203	237	J09(RS2), D00, D01, D04
2. Causes of orantral fistula.	208	242	J14(RS2)
CHAPTER 35 ANATOMY AND PHYSIOLOGY OF PARANASAL SINUSES			
Long Essay			
1. Describe the anatomy and functions of paranasal sinuses.	209	176, 182	J09(RS2)
Short Answer			
1. Sphenoid sinus.	210	178	J08(RS2)
CHAPTER 36 ACUTE SINUSITIS			
Long Essay			
1. Acute maxillary sinusitis—etiopathology, clinical features, investigations and treatment.	214	201	D18(RS3)
Short Essay			
1. Management of acute maxillary sinusitis.	215	203	J14
Short Answer			
1. Treatment of acute frontal sinusitis.	215	203	D13
CHAPTER 37 CHRONIC SINUSITIS			
Long Essay			
1. Chronic frontal and maxillary sinusitis—etiopathology, clinical features and management.	217	204	D16

Contd...

Contd...

	DNGR	BNSL	
CHAPTER 44 **TUMORS OF ORAL CAVITY**			
Short Essays			
1. Premalignant conditions of the oral cavity.	253	264	D19(RS3), D14
2. Leukoplakia.	253	264	D12
3. Discuss etiology of oral malignancies.	254	282	J08
Short Answers			
1. Ranula.	252	282	J11(RS2), D11(RS2), D16(RS3), J14
2. Premalignant conditions of oral cavity.	253	264	D07(RS2), J10
3. Leukoplakia (of oral cavity/tongue).	253	264	D17(RS3), D00, J02, D04, J07
CHAPTER 45 **NON-NEOPLASTIC DISORDERS OF SALIVARY GLANDS**			
Short Essay			
1. Sialolithiasis—management.	261	274	D05
Short Answers			
1. Acute parotitis.	259	272	J19(RS3)
2. Submandibular salivary calculus.	260	274	D01
3. Treatment of salivary calculi.	261	274	J17(RS3)
CHAPTER 46 **NEOPLASMS OF SALIVARY GLANDS**			
Short Essay			
1. Parotid neoplasms.	263	275	D14(RS3)
Short Answer			
1. Pleomorphic adenoma (clinical features).	263	275	D13(RS2), D06

Contd...

Contd...

	DNGR	BNSL	
Section IV: Diseases of Pharynx			
CHAPTER 47 ANATOMY AND PHYSIOLOGY OF PHARYNX			
Short Essays			
1. Describe in detail the surgical approaches to nasopharynx.	—	—	J17(RS3)
2. What are the differences between tonsils and adenoids?	—	291	J03
3. Killian's dehiscence.	269	289	D11
4. What is Killian's dehiscence? Discuss management of pharyngeal pouch.	269, 311	289	J14(RS2)
5. Waldeyer's ring and its importance.	269	289	J15(RS3), D19(RS3), J03
6. Pyriform fossa.	272	294	J09(RS2)
Short Answers			
1. Killian's dehiscence.	269	289	D11(RS2)
2. Waldeyer's ring.	269	289	D09(RS2), J11(RS2), D12(RS3), D13(RS2), D16(RS3), D08, J10
3. Fossa of Rosenmuller.	270	290	D14(RS3)
4. Sinus of Morgagni	271	290	D14
5. Pyriform sinus (fossa).	272	294	J15(RS3), D15(RS3), D19(RS3)
CHAPTER 48 ADENOIDS AND OTHER INFLAMMATIONS OF NASOPHARYNX			
Short Essays			
1. Adenoiditis—etiology, clinical features and management.	275	308	J16(RS3), J04
2. Adenoid facies.	275	308	D11(RS2), D02

Contd...

OTORHINOLARYNGOLOGY

Contd...

	DNGR	BNSL	
Short Answer			
1. Adenoid facies.	275	308	J12(RS2), J13(RS3), J14(RS2), D10, J14, J17

CHAPTER 49
TUMORS OF NASOPHARYNX

	DNGR	BNSL	
Long Essays			
1. Juvenile nasopharyngeal angiofibroma (JNA)—etiopathology, clinical features, diagnosis and management.	279	317	D09(RS2), J11(RS2), D16(RS3), J01, D01, D08, D14
2. Carcinoma nasopharynx—etiopathology, clinical features and management.	283	320	J08(RS2)
Short Essays			
1. Juvenile nasopharyngeal angiofibroma (JNA)—clinical features, diagnosis, management.	279	317	D10(RS2), D12(RS3), J15(RS3), J04, D05, J09, D12
2. Carcinoma nasopharynx—management.	283	320	J06, D06

CHAPTER 50
ACUTE AND CHRONIC PHARYNGITIS

	DNGR	BNSL	
Short Essays			
1. Tonsillar keratosis.	280	307	D00
2. Keratosis pharyngitis.	289	307	J06
Short Answers			
1. Hyperkeratosis of tonsil.	289	307	D10
2. Keratosis pharyngis.	289	307	D15(RS3)

Contd...

Contd...

	DNGR	BNSL	
CHAPTER 51 **ACUTE AND CHRONIC TONSILLITIS**			
Long Essays			
1. Enumerate the conditions causing patch on the tonsils and their management.	293	305	D02, D04
2. Chronic tonsillitis—types, clinicopathological features and management.	294	304	J10
Short Essays			
1. Anatomy of palatine tonsil.	291	292	D15
2. Acute tonsillitis—clinical features and management.	292	304	D12
3. Membranous tonsillitis.	293	305	J10(RS2)
4. Differential diagnosis (causes) of a white patch (membrane) on the tonsil.	293	305	D11(RS2), J16(RS3), J17(RS3), J04, J06, J07
5. How would you diagnose and treat tonsillar diphtheria?	293	306	D10
6. Faucial diphtheria.	294	306	D19(RS3)
7. Chronic tonsillitis—clinical features (cardinal signs) and management.	294	308	D06, D13
Short Answers			
1. Anatomy of palatine tonsil.	291	292	D06
2. Lateral relations of tonsils.	291	292	D11
3. Differences between palatine tonsil and lymph node.	—	—	J06
4. Blood supply of palatine tonsil.	291	293	D09(RS2), D11(RS2), D07, J12, D12
5. Membranous conditions of tonsil.	293	305	D07(RS2)
6. Types of chronic tonsillitis.	294	—	D19(RS3)
7. Cardinal signs of chronic tonsillitis.	295	308	J15(RS3), J16(RS3), D18(RS3), J19(RS3), D05

Contd...

Contd...

		DNGR	BNSL	
8.	Enumerate complications of chronic tonsillitis.	295	308	D14
9.	Tonsillolith.	295	307	D17(RS3), J13
10.	Lingual tonsillitis.	295	307	D02, J05

CHAPTER 52
HEAD AND NECK SPACE INFECTIONS

Long Essays

1.	Enumerate the ENT conditions presenting with trismus. Discuss the etiopathology, clinical features and management of peritonsillar abscess (quinsy).	435, 298	430, 427	D03, J17
2.	Discuss the etiopathology, clinical features and management of deep neck space infections.	299	428	D09(RS2)
3.	Describe the anatomy of retro pharyngeal space. Discuss the etiopathogenesis, clinical features and management of (acute) retropharyngeal abscess.	299	426, 428	D14(RS3), J07
4.	Name the two types of retropharyngeal abscess. Describe the etiology, pathogenesis, clinical features and treatment of any one of them.	300	428	D00

Short Essays

1.	Ludwig's angina.	297	429	D11(RS2), D15(RS3), D17(RS3), J01, J13
2.	Peritonsillar abscess (quinsy)—define, etiopathogenesis, clinical features and management.	298	427	J11(RS2), J14(RS2), D15(RS3), D16(RS3), D18(RS3), J01, D01, J02, J08, D08, D10, J12

Contd...

Contd...

		DNGR	BNSL	
3.	Retropharyngeal abscess—etiology and management.	299	428	J08(RS2), J14(RS2), J09
4.	Acute retropharyngeal abscess—etiology, clinical features and management.	300	428	D13(RS2), D08, D11, J12
5.	Chronic retropharyngeal abscess.	301	429	J16(RS3), J18(RS3), D02
6.	Tuberculous cervical lymphadenitis.	—	415	J07, J14
7.	Parapharyngeal space (anatomy and its surgical approaches).	301	426	J17(RS3), J19(RS3)
8.	Parapharyngeal space abscess.	301	428	D14, D15
Short Answers				
1.	Ludwig's angina.	297	429	D10(RS2), J16(RS3), J17(RS3), D05, J09
2.	Peritonsillar abscess (quinsy).	298	427	D07(RS2), J16, D16
3.	Space of Gillette.	299	426	D01, J02, J05
4.	Acute retropharyngeal abscess.	300	428	D16
5.	Parapharyngeal space.	301	426	D12(RS3), J03
6.	Parapharyngeal abscess.	301	428	J10

CHAPTER 53
TUMORS OF OROPHARYNX

Short Essays				
1.	Etiology of oropharyngeal cancer.	—	325	J08(RS2)
2.	Eagle's syndrome.	308	329	J10(RS2), D08
Short Answer				
1.	Elongated styloid process (Eagle's syndrome).	308	329	D14(RS3), J02, D11

Contd...

Contd...

	DNGR	BNSL	
CHAPTER 54 **TUMORS OF THE HYPOPHARYNX AND PHARYNGEAL POUCH**			
Short Essay			
1. Post-cricoid malignancy.	309	332	J08(RS2)
CHAPTER 55 **SNORING AND SLEEP APNEA**			
Short Essay			
1. Obstructive sleep apnea syndrome.	313	311	J10(RS2), D10(RS2), D12(RS3), D14(RS3), J17
Short Answer			
1. Sleep apnea	313	311	D09(RS2), J13

Section V: Diseases of Larynx and Trachea

	DNGR	BNSL	
CHAPTER 56 **ANATOMY AND PHYSIOLOGY OF LARYNX**			
Long Essay			
1. Discuss the physiology of phonation.	323	352	J08(RS2)
Short Essays			
1. Intrinsic muscles of larynx.	320	349	J08(RS2)
2. Differences between adult and infant's larynx.	323	—	J09(RS2), D11(RS2), D15
3. Functions of larynx.	323	352	D12(RS3)
Short Answers			
1. Laryngeal cartilages (mention)—unpaired cartilages.	319	346	J09(RS2), D18(RS3), D11
2. Thyroid cartilage.	319	346	D01, J05
3. Cricovocal membrane.	320	347	D14
4. Laryngeal ventricle.	321	348	J02

Contd...

Contd...

		DNGR	BNSL	
5.	Differences between adult and infant larynx.	323	—	D10(RS2)
6.	Functions of larynx.	323	352	J10(RS2), D14

CHAPTER 57
LARYNGOTRACHEAL TRAUMA

Long Essay

1.	Discuss the etiopathology, clinical features and management of laryngotracheal trauma.	325	400	D15(RS3)

CHAPTER 58
ACUTE AND CHRONIC INFLAMMATIONS OF LARYNX

Short Essays

1.	Acute epiglotitis (clinical features and management).	327	362	J08(RS2), D17(RS3), D12
2.	Laryngeal diphtheria.	328	363	D14
3.	Tuberculosis of larynx.	331	365	J15

Short Answers

1.	Epiglottitis in children.	327	362	D00, D04
2.	Acute epiglottitis (management).	327	362	D14(RS3), J18(RS3)
3.	Reinke's edema.	330	369	J10(RS2), J11(RS2), D16(RS3), D19(RS3), D14
4.	Tuberculosis of larynx—clinical features.	331	365	D18(RS3), J09

CHAPTER 59
CONGENITAL LESIONS OF LARYNX AND STRIDOR

Long Essays

1.	Define stridor. Enumerate the causes of stridor. How do you manage a patient of stridor?	333	358	J16(RS3), J03, J11

Contd...

Contd...

	DNGR	BNSL	
2. Classify the causes of stridor in a child. Discuss the clinical features and management of juvenile laryngeal papillomatosis.	334, 345	358, 371	D05
Short Essays			
1. Laryngomalacia (congenital laryngeal stridor).	333	396	D09(RS2), J14
2. Subglottic stenosis.	333	397	J17
3. Stridor—define, causes (in children).	333	358	J14(RS2), D19(RS3), D00, D04, J16
Short Answers			
1. Laryngomalacia.	333	396	D15(RS3), J18(RS3), J07, J12
2. Subglottic stenosis.	333	397	J01
3. Laryngeal web.	333	397	J16(RS3), D02, J05, J16
4. Stridor (etiology in children).	333	358	J12(RS2), J13(RS3), D13(RS2), J15(RS3)
5. Enumerate causes of congenital laryngeal stridor.	334	358	J10

CHAPTER 60
LARYNGEAL PARALYSIS

Short Essays			
1. Difference between the right and left recurrent laryngeal nerve anatomy.	—	350	J05
2. Nerve supply of larynx.	337	350	D15(RS3)
3. Enumerate the causes of vocal cord paralysis. How do you investigate and manage a case of unilateral vocal cord paralysis.	337	375	J02, D04
4. Causes of left recurrent laryngeal nerve paralysis.	337	375	D06

Contd...

Contd...

	DNGR	BNSL	
Short Answers			
1. Causes of left vocal cord paralysis.	337	375	J17
2. Recurrent laryngeal nerve.	337	350	D09(RS2)
3. Bilateral adductor paralysis.	338	376	J10(RS2)

CHAPTER 61
BENIGN TUMORS OF LARYNX

	DNGR	BNSL	
Long Essay			
1. Juvenile laryngeal papilloma—etiopathology, clinical features, management and complications.	345	371	J15(RS3)
Short Essays			
1. Singer's nodule (vocal nodule).	343	368	J16(RS3), J04, J07, D08, D10, D13
2. Vocal polyp (etiopathology and management).	343	369	J06
3. Laryngocele.	345	371	D01, J05, J07, J12
4. Papillomas of larynx.	345	371	D07(RS2)
5. Juvenile laryngeal papillomatosis.	345	371	D17(RS3), D13
6. Multiple papillomas of larynx.	345	371	J08
Short Answers			
1. Premalignant lesions of larynx.	—	370	J14(RS2)
2. Vocal nodule (Singer's nodule/laryngeal nodules)—management.	343	368	J14(RS2), D14(RS3), D17(RS3), J01, D01, D03, J08, D12, J13, D15, J17
3. Vocal cord polyps.	343	369	J08(RS2), J11(RS2), D12(RS3), D16(RS3), J10
4. Laryngocele.	345	371	D17(RS3), J19(RS3)
5. Laryngeal papilloma.	345	371	J15(RS3)

Contd...

Contd...

	DNGR	BNSL	
CHAPTER 62			
CANCER LARYNX			
Long Essay			
1. Carcinoma larynx—etiology, symptoms, signs, investigations and treatment.	347	382	D10(RS2)
Short Essays			
1. Pharyngo-cutaneous fistula.	—	—	J08(RS2)
2. Glottic cancers have high cure rate. Give reasons.	—	—	D00, J03, D04
3. TNM classification of carcinoma of glottis.	348	385	J15
4. Investigations and treatment of glottic cancer.	350	383	J04
5. How do you manage a stage III carcinoma larynx?	351	384	D07(RS2)
6. Speech rehabilitation following laryngectomy.	352	387	D05
Short Answers			
1. TNM classification of carcinoma larynx.	348	385	D07
2. T1 glottic malignancy.	348	385	D03
3. Esophageal voice.	352	388	D00, D02, D04, J05
CHAPTER 63			
VOICE AND SPEECH DISORDERS			
Short Essays			
1. Discuss the management of an adult patient presenting with hoarseness of voice.	—	—	J17(RS3)
2. 'Hoarse voice'—causes (in a 55 year-old-male).	355	357	D07(RS2), D13
3. Functional aphonia.	356	379	D05, D11
4. Rhinolalia.	357	380	J10
Short Answers			
1. Enumerate causes of hoarseness in a 50-year-old female.	355	357	J10

Contd...

Contd...

		DNGR	BNSL	
2.	Puberphonia.	356	380	D09(RS2), J11, J15
3.	Rhinolalia.	357	380	D08(RS2)
4.	Rhinolalia aperta (causes).	357	380	D01, J02
5.	Rhinolalia clausa.	357	380	J03, J16

CHAPTER 64
TRACHEOSTOMY AND OTHER PROCEDURES FOR AIRWAY MANAGEMENT

Long Essay

1.	What is stridor? Describe briefly the indications, procedure and complications of tracheostomy.	333, 360	358, 390	J19(RS3)

Short Essays

1.	Advantages of tracheostomy over endotracheal intubation.	—	—	D06
2.	Tracheostomy—types, indications (nonobstructive), procedure and complications.	359	390	D07(RS2), D08(RS2), J11(RS2), D12(RS3), J15(RS3), D16(RS3), J17(RS3), J04, D04, J08, J10, D14, J17
3.	Postoperative care/management after tracheostomy.	361	393	J18(RS3)
4.	What is emergency tracheostomy? Name the indications for it.	363	391	D02

Short Answers

1.	Indications for tracheostomy.	360	390	D10(RS2), J12
2.	Nonobstructive indication for tracheostomy.	360	390	D15
3.	Decannulation of tracheostomy.	361	393	D11
4.	Causes of decannulation problem.	361	393	D03
5.	Complications of tracheostomy.	362	393	D05, J08, J16

Contd...

Contd...

	DNGR	BNSL	
Short Answers			
1. Foreign body in cricopharynx.	395	—	D10
2. Foreign body esophagus.	395	337	D01
3. Management of ingested foreign body.	396	338	J06
Section VIII: Recent Advances			
CHAPTER 71 **LASER SURGERY, RADIOFREQUENCY SURGERY, HYPERBARIC OXYGEN THERAPY AND COBLATION**			
Short Answer			
1. Laser—define, types, applications in ENT.	401	492	D10(RS2), J14(RS2), D18(RS3), J09
CHAPTER 72 **CRYOSURGERY**			
Short Essay			
1. Cryosurgery in otorhinolaryngology.	409	496	J12
CHAPTER 73 **RADIOTHERAPY IN HEAD AND NECK CANCER**			
Short Answer			
1. Enumerate complications of radiotherapy.	418	487	J09
CHAPTER 74 **CHEMOTHERAPY IN HEAD AND NECK CANCER**			
Short Answers			
1. Chemotherapy.	419	488	D08(RS2)
2. Palliative treatment.	419	490	D08(RS2)
CHAPTER 75 **HIV INFECTIONS/AIDS AND ENT MANIFESTATIONS**			
Short Essay			
1. Manifestation of acquired immunodeficiency syndrome (AIDS) in ENT.	422	500	D07(RS2), D13

Contd...

OTORHINOLARYNGOLOGY

Contd...

	DNGR	BNSL	
Short Answer			
1. ENT manifestations in acquired immunodeficiency syndrome.	422	500	D10(RS2)

Section IX: Clinical Methods in ENT and Neck Masses

CHAPTER 76 CLINICAL METHODS IN ENT

Short Essay			
1. Enumerate cause of trismus. Discuss management of one common cause.	435	430	D07
Short Answers			
1. Uses of Siegle's pneumatic aural speculum.	430	464	J08
2. Anterior rhinoscopy.	431	186	J10(RS2)
3. Posterior rhinoscopy (diagram of structures seen).	432	186	J18(RS3), D19(RS3), J14, D15
4. Enumerate causes of trismus.	435	430	D15(RS3), D08
5. Laryngeal crepitus.	437	—	J08
6. Indirect laryngoscopy (diagrammatic view of structures seen).	437	355	D15(RS3), D00, D02, D04, D13, J16

CHAPTER 77 NECK MASSES

Short Essays			
1. Give differential diagnosis of lymph node in neck.	—	—	J08
2. Differential diagnosis of a midline neck swelling.	445	—	D12(RS3), D13(RS2), D14(RS3)
3. Thyroglossal cyst.	445	414	J12(RS2), J13(RS3), D18(RS3), J19(RS3), D01, D02, D13

Contd...

Contd...

	DNGR	BNSL	
4. Differential diagnosis of lateral neck swellings.	446	—	J11(RS2), D16(RS3)
5. Branchial cyst.	446	414	D18(RS3), J13
Short Answers			
1. Causes of midline neck swelling.	445	—	D19(RS3)
2. Thyroglossal cyst.	445	414	D15(RS3), J09
3. Branchial cyst.	446	414	J11(RS2), D16(RS3)
4. Plunging ranula.	447	282	D14(RS3)

Section X: Operative Surgery

CHAPTER 78 MYRINGOTOMY

Short Essay

1. Myringotomy—indications, procedure and complications.	453	432	J02, D07
Short Answers			
1. Indications for gromet insertion in ear.	453	432	J05
2. Myringotomy (indications and sites).	453	432	D07(RS2), D18(RS3), J14

CHAPTER 79 EAR SURGERY AND APPROACHES

Short Answer

1. Describe the types of mastoidectomies.	455	433	J03

CHAPTER 80 CORTICAL MASTOIDECTOMY

Short Essay

1. Define coalescent mastoiditis. Describe cortical mastoidectomy.	84, 457	119, 434	J12(RS2), J13(RS3), D12

Contd...

Contd...

	DNGR	BNSL	
Short Answers			
1. Simple mastoidectomy.	457	434	D15
2. Complications of mastoidectomy.	458	436	J09(RS2), J13

CHAPTER 81
RADICAL MASTOIDECTOMY

None

CHAPTER 82
MODIFIED RADICAL MASTOIDECTOMY

Short Answer			
1. Modified radical mastoidectomy	461	437	D16

CHAPTER 83
MYRINGOPLASTY

Short Essay			
1. Myringoplasty	463	439	D10
Short Answers			
1. Myringoplasty	463	439	J09
2. Graft materials for Myringoplasty	463	439	J17

CHAPTER 84
PROOF PUNCTURE (ANTRAL IRRIGATION)

Short Essay			
1. Antral lavage/Antral wash.	465	444	D07(RS2), J12, D15
Short Answer			
1. Antral puncture (indications and complications).	465	444	D07

CHAPTER 85
INTRANASAL INFERIOR MEATAL ANTROSTOMY

None

Contd...

Contd...

	DNGR	BNSL	
CHAPTER 86 **CALDWELL-LUC OPERATION**			
Short Essay			
1. Caldwell-Luc's operation—indications, procedure (steps) and complications.	469	445	J19(RS3), J03, J08
Short Answer			
1. Caldwell-Luc operation—indications.	469	445	J17(RS3), D08, D13
CHAPTER 87 **SUBMUCOUS RESECTION OF NASAL SEPTUM (SMR OPERATION)**			
Short Essays			
1. Discuss the difference between septoplasty and submucous resection of nasal septum (SMR) operation.	—	447	J10(RS2), J19(RS3), D00, J01, D04, D05, J13, D14
2. Submucous resection (SMR) of nasal septum—indications and complications.	471	447	D03, J08, J16
3. Discuss complications and their management of nasal septal surgery. Describe septal abscess.	471, 473, 168	449, 232	D10
Short Answer			
1. Submucous resection of nasal septum (indications/complications).	471	447	J08(RS2), J10
CHAPTER 88 **SEPTOPLASTY**			
Short Answer			
1. Septoplasty.	473	447	D16
CHAPTER 89 **DIAGNOSTIC NASAL ENDOSCOPY**			
Short Answer			
1. Diagnostic nasal endoscopy (technique).	475	441	J09(RS2), D10(RS2), J14

Contd...

Contd...

	DNGR	BNSL	
CHAPTER 90 **ENDOSCOPIC SINUS SURGERY**			
Short Essay			
1. Endoscopic sinus surgery.	477	442	J16(RS3)
CHAPTER 91 **DIRECT LARYNGOSCOPY**			
Short Essay			
1. Rigid (direct) laryngoscopy—indications and contraindications.	481	456	D19(RS3), J01, J03
Short Answer			
1. Indications for direct laryngoscopy.	481	456	J05
CHAPTER 92 **BRONCHOSCOPY**			
Short Essay			
1. (Rigid) bronchoscopy (Indications, contraindications and complications).	483	458	D11(RS2), J17(RS3), D03, D12
CHAPTER 93 **ESOPHAGOSCOPY**			
Short Essay			
1. (Rigid) esophagoscopy (indications, contraindications and complications).	485	459	J12(RS2), J13(RS3), D13(RS2), J04, J11, J15, D16
Short Answer			
1. Esophagoscopy (complications).	485	459	J06, J11
CHAPTER 94 **TONSILLECTOMY**			
Short Essays			
1. Tonsillectomy—indications and complications.	487	450	D10(RS2), D13(RS2), J07, J13, J14, D15

Contd...

Contd...

	DNGR	BNSL	
2. Briefly describe the operative steps of dissection method of tonsillectomy.	487	452	J06
3. Secondary hemorrhage.	490	454	J15(RS3)
Short Answers			
1. Absolute contraindications for tonsillectomy.	487	451	J18(RS3)
2. Enumerate the complications of tonsillitis.	489	454	J14
3. Immediate complications of tonsillectomy.	489	454	J17
4. Reactionary hemorrhage after tonsillectomy.	489	454	D00, J01, D04
5. Management of reactionary hemorrhage following tonsillectomy.	489	454	J14(RS2)
6. Secondary hemorrhage following tonsillectomy—causes and treatment.	490	454	D07

CHAPTER 95
ADENOIDECTOMY

Short Essay			
1. Adenoidectomy (indications and complications).	491	451	D14(RS3), J09
Short Answers			
1. Complications of adenoidectomy.	491	454	D06
2. Post-adenoidectomy hemorrhage.	491	454	J02

CHAPTER 96
RADIOLOGY IN ENT

Short Answer			
1. X-ray PNS.	493	476	J18(RS3)

MISCELLANEOUS

Short Essays			
1. Tracheostomy tubes.	524	472	J16(RS3), D01, J05, J13
2. Describe features of ideal tracheostomy tube.	—	472	D07

Contd...

OTORHINOLARYNGOLOGY

Contd...

		DNGR	BNSL	
3.	Glandular fever.	—	—	J15(RS3)
4.	Write a note on microlaryngeal surgery (MLS).	—	378	D00, J01, D04
5.	What are the causes of unilateral nasal discharge?	—	—	J02, J08
6.	Give the differential diagnosis of unilateral nasal mass.	—	188	J04
7.	Mention the branches of external carotid artery.	—	—	J05
8.	Indications and technique of microlaryngoscopy.	—	378	J06
9.	TNM staging and its clinical application.	—	—	J08(RS2)
10.	Bronchopulmonary segments.	—	—	J08(RS2)
11.	Precancerous conditions in ENT.	—	—	J18(RS3), J11
12.	Anaerobic infection in ENT.	—	—	J09(RS2)
13.	Occult primary.	—	—	J09
14.	Role of local anesthesia in oto-rhino-laryngology.	—	—	D08(RS2)
15.	Nasal decongestants.	—	—	D08(RS2)
16.	Newer generation antihistaminics.	—	—	J09(RS2)
17.	Dangerous area of the face.	—	—	J12(RS2), J13(RS3)
Short Answers				
1.	Battle's sign.	507	—	D11
2.	Thornwaldt's cyst.	510	291	J15
3.	Sluder's neuralgia.	510	221	D11
4.	Tracheostomy tubes—types, its advantages and disadvantages.	524	472	D11(RS2), D14(RS3), J18(RS3)
5.	Symptoms of nasal disease.	—	185	D16
6.	Symptoms of laryngeal diseases.	—	355	D16
7.	Six causes of reddish mass in right nasal cavity.	—	188	D06
8.	Prevention of Iatrogenic laryngotracheal stenosis.	—	—	J06

Contd...

Contd...

		DNGR	BNSL	
9.	External carotid artery branches.	—	—	J09(RS2), D10
10.	Carcinoma in-situ.	—	—	D09(RS2)
11.	Post-nasal drip.	—	—	J10(RS2)
12.	Mucociliary dyskinesia.	—	—	D10(RS2)
13.	Cardiospasm.	—	—	D10
14.	Compare indirect and direct laryngoscopy.	—	—	D10
15.	Nasal decongestants.		—	D11(RS2)
16.	Cold abscess of neck.		—	D12(RS3)
17.	Leukotriene inhibitors.		—	D12

EU GSPR Authorised Reprsentative
Logos Europe, 9 rue Nicolas Poussin
1700, La Rochelle, France
Phone: +33 (0) 6 67 93 73 78
E-mail: contact@logoseurope.eu

www.ingramcontent.com/pod-product-compliance
Ingram Content Group UK Ltd.
Pitfield, Milton Keynes, MK11 3LW, UK
UKHW020732210726
13898UKWH00025B/639
9789389776508